100 Questions & Answers About Vulvar Cancer and Other Diseases of the Vulva and the Vagina

Lara J. Burrows, MD, MSC

The Center for Vulvovaginal Disorders
Washington, DC

Debra S. Heller, MD

Professor of Pathology & Laboratory Medicine
Professor of Obstetrics, Gynecology, & Women's Health
UMDNJ-New Jersey Medical School
Newark, New Jersey

JONES AND BARTLETT PUBLISHERS
Sudbury, Massachusetts
BOSTON TORONTO LONDON SINGAPORE

World Headquarters
Jones and Bartlett Publishers
40 Tall Pine Drive
Sudbury, MA 01776
978-443-5000
info@jbpub.com
www.jbpub.com

Jones and Bartlett Publishers
Canada
6339 Ormindale Way
Mississauga, Ontario L5V 1J2
Canada

Jones and Bartlett Publishers
International
Barb House, Barb Mews
London W6 7PA
United Kingdom

Jones and Bartlett's books and products are available through most bookstores and online booksellers. To contact Jones and Bartlett Publishers directly, call 800-832-0034, fax 978-443-8000, or visit our website, www.jbpub.com.

Substantial discounts on bulk quantities of Jones and Bartlett's publications are available to corporations, professional associations, and other qualified organizations. For details and specific discount information, contact the special sales department at Jones and Bartlett via the above contact information or send an email to specialsales@jbpub.com.

The authors, editor, and publisher have made every effort to provide accurate information. However, they are not responsible for errors, omissions, or for any outcomes related to the use of the contents of this book and take no responsibility for the use of the products and procedures described. Treatments and side effects described in this book may not be applicable to all people; likewise, some people may require a dose or experience a side effect that is not described herein. Drugs and medical devices are discussed that may have limited availability controlled by the Food and Drug Administration (FDA) for use only in a research study or clinical trial. Research, clinical practice, and government regulations often change the accepted standard in this field. When consideration is being given to use of any drug in the clinical setting, the healthcare provider or reader is responsible for determining FDA status of the drug, reading the package insert, and reviewing prescribing information for the most up-to-date recommendations on dose, precautions, and contraindications, and determining the appropriate usage for the product. This is especially important in the case of drugs that are new or seldom used.

Production Credits

Executive Publisher: Christopher Davis
Custom Projects Editor: Kathy Richardson
Senior Editorial Assistant: Jessica Acox
Production Assistant: Ashlee Hazeltine
Marketing Manager: Ilana Goddess
V.P. of Manufacturing and Inventory Control: Therese Connell
Composition: Spoke & Wheel/Jason Miranda
Cover Design: Carolyn Downer
Cover Image: Top: © Monkey Business Images/ShutterStock, Inc.; Bottom Left: © Konstantin Chagin/ShutterStock, Inc.; Bottom Right: © Photodisc/Alamy Images
Printing and Binding: Malloy, Inc.
Cover Printing: Malloy, Inc.

Library of Congress Cataloging-in-Publication Data

Burrows, Lara.
100 questions and answers about vulvar cancer and other diseases of the vulva and the vagina / Lara Burrows and Debra Heller.
p. cm.
Includes index.
ISBN-13: 978-0-7637-5825-7 (pbk.)
ISBN-10: 0-7637-5825-6 (ibid)
1. Vulva—Cancer—Popular works. 2. Vulva—Cancer—Miscellanea. 3. Vulva—Diseases—Miscellanea. 4. Vagina—Diseases—Miscellanea. I. Heller, Debra S. II. Title. III. Title: One hundred questions and answers about vulvar cancer and other diseases of the vulva and the vagina.
RC280.V8B87 2009
618.1'6—dc22

2008044990

6048

Printed in the United States of America
13 12 11 10 09 10 9 8 7 6 5 4 3 2 1

To my husband, Hooman, whose infinite patience makes all of my projects possible and to my mentor Andrew, whose creativity nurtures my projects to fruition.

Lara J. Burrows, MD, MSC

To Cardie, Cathy B., Cathy R., Ann Marie, Lynne, and Val. Family comes in many forms.

Debra S. Heller, MD

CONTENTS

PREFACE

The vulva is thought of in many ways, if it is thought of at all. The art of Georgia O'Keefe is thought to celebrate the beauty of that part of the female anatomy. To some, the vulva is a mysterious place, "down there," never to be referred to by its correct name. The vulva is both an organ composed of skin and a gynecologic organ. Because of this, the vulva is prone to both skin diseases one can get anywhere on the body and unique problems that can only affect the vulva. These problems can sometimes be prevented by appropriate hygiene and care, and can always be treated with the hopes of curing or at least improving the condition. Vulvar problems can sometimes cause a great deal of discomfort and worry for the affected woman, made worse, perhaps, because it is "down there," in an area rarely discussed. Our hope in writing this book is to make an area of the body thought mysterious by some, less so. We hope this will help women be their own advocates, and help them in their conversations with their medical care providers. While we may never eradicate the concept of "down there," perhaps we can make the vulva a less mysterious area of the body.

PART ONE

The Basics

What is "down there"? What is the vulva?

I have little bumps on my labia minora. Does this mean I have warts?

What does it mean when the vagina has an odor?

More . . .

Uterus

The female womb.

Ovaries

The female gonad or reproductive gland, in which the ova and the hormones that regulate female secondary sex characteristics develop.

Fallopian tubes

A pair of long, slender ducts in the female abdomen that transport ova from the ovary to the uterus and, in fertilization, transport sperm cells from the uterus to the released egg.

Vagina

The passage leading from the uterus to the vulva in women.

Vulva

A woman's external genitalia. The vulva includes the mons pubis, the clitoris, the inner labia minora (small lips) and labia majora (large lips), and the opening to the vagina (but not the vaginal canal itself), called the vulvar vestibule.

1. What is "down there"? What is the vulva?

Female genital anatomy can be thought of as having an internal part (the inside that we can't see) and an external part (the outside that we can see). The internal organs are the **uterus** (also called the womb), the **ovaries** (which make the eggs), the **fallopian tubes** (where fertilization occurs), and the **vagina** (the birth canal). The vagina is a *potential* space; it is not always open, but is rather more like a balloon that can expand when something is inside (e.g., tampon and penis). During daily activities, the walls of the vagina touch each other from front to back, and the space is closed.

The **vulva** refers to a woman's external genitalia. Although you may have heard this part of the body referred to as the vagina, this is not technically correct. There are also many slang terms for the vulva. The vulva includes the **mons pubis**, which is the soft, fatty pad of tissue covering the pubic bone on which pubic hair starts to grow during puberty, the **clitoris**, which is located at the upper joining of the **labia minora**, the inner labia minora (small lips) and **labia majora** (large lips), and the opening to the vagina (but not the vaginal canal itself), called the **vulvar vestibule**. The labia majora are two fat pads that are typically covered with pubic hair-bearing skin after puberty. Between the labia majora are the labia minora, which are two folds of tissue that meet at the sensitive **clitoral hood** (**Figure 1**). There are four openings within the vulvar vestibule: the vagina, the **urethra**, and the two **Bartholin's gland** duct openings. The urethra is the tube exiting the bladder, from which urine is passed.

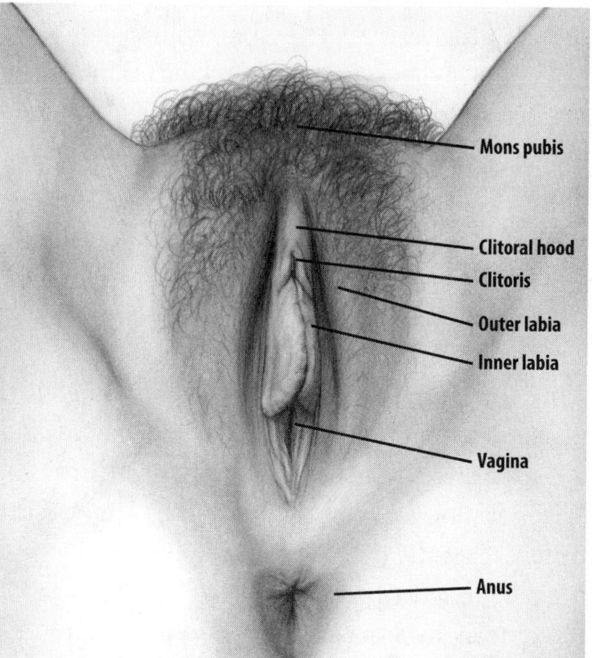

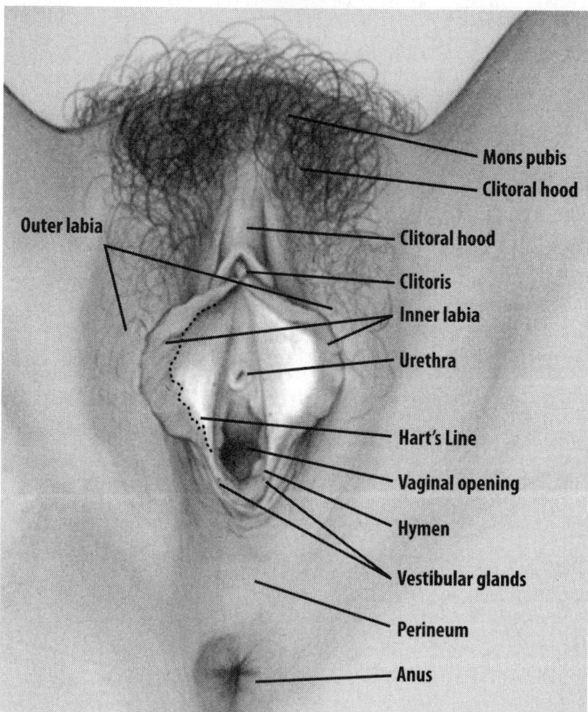

Figure 1 The normal vulva.

Mons pubis

A rounded fleshy protuberance situated over the pubic bones that becomes covered with hair during puberty.

Clitoris

The erectile organ of the female vulva, homologous to the penis of the male.

Labia minora (small lips)

These are two folds of tissue that meet at the sensitive clitoral hood.

Labia majora (large lips)

Two fat pads that are typically covered with pubic hair-bearing skin after puberty. Between the labia majora is the labia minora.

Vulvar vestibule

A part of the vulva between the labia minora that the urethral opening and the vaginal opening.

Clitoral hood

A protective hood of tissue that covers the clitoris.

Urethra

The canal through which urine is discharged from the bladder.

Bartholin's glands

Paired glands at the 4- and 8-o'clock positions at the vaginal opening. Sometimes they can become infected and form a painful abscess.

Menopause

The decrease of estrogen levels in women. A variety of changes may occur including thinning of the vulvar skin. The vulvar skin is sensitive to the effects of estrogen and without it becomes delicate, thin, dry, and sometimes more sensitive.

It is at the top of the vestibule. The Bartholin's glands are paired structures at the 4- and 8-o'clock positions of the vestibule, and their ducts exit at those positions. The Bartholin's glands provide lubrication during sexual arousal. The vestibule is also the entranceway to the vagina.

The vulva changes in appearance over the course of a woman's life. The labia are smaller, and there is no hair in the prepubertal child. Estrogen leads to an increase in size, making the vulva look fatter. Public hair and labial size decrease after **menopause**. The labia majora and minora are sexually responsive and swell during arousal. The clitoris is analogous to the penis and becomes erect during arousal. It is the main site for the female orgasm, and a large percentage of women require direct stimulation of the clitoris in order to have an orgasm, not climaxing from intercourse alone.

2. How should I care for my vulva and vagina?

The dictum "less is more" applies to the best way to care for the vulva. Women's bodies are designed to do most of the work. The skin of the vulva is very delicate and sensitive and can become more so after menopause. Normal secretions from the vagina help to keep the vagina clean and healthy. Using chemicals, soaps, shower gels, and "feminine wipes"; washing too often (more than once a day); and rubbing too hard when drying the area can irritate this delicate area or cause an allergic response. The use of a gentle, mild, nonscented soap with plain, lukewarm water is best. If there is sensitivity, warm water alone is even better.

Tight pants, pantyhose, and thongs may irritate the vulva. Cotton undergarments that are washed in a mild detergent are the least irritating. Feminine pads should be nonscented, and the best ones are 100% cotton and hypoallergenic. White unscented toilet paper is best.

Additional patient information on the normal vulva and vulvar hygiene, as well as on a variety of medical conditions, can be accessed from the International Society for the Study of Vulvovaginal Diseases at *www.ISSVD.org* (**Tables 1** and **2**).

Additional patient information on the vulva can be accessed from the International Society for the Study of Vulvovaginal Diseases at www.ISSVD.org.

The vagina does not need to be washed; it is "self-cleaning" from the production of normal secretions. It is normal for the vulvovaginal area to have a light scent. If the smell is particularly strong or fish-like, then a health professional should be consulted to rule out **vaginitis** or other conditions. The healthy vagina contains **bacteria**, just as our mouths do. This is normal and is not considered to be an infection. These bacteria maintain an "acidic" environment in the vagina, which helps to prevent bacterial or **yeast infections**. Douching is not recommended, as it can wash away these good bacteria, leading to irritation and infection with an overgrowth of "bad" organisms. Also, some women may be allergic to various douching products. Women who have a specific problem in this area may be prescribed creams or gels and occasionally medicinal douches; however, a health care provider should supervise this.

Vaginitis

Inflammation of the vagina. It may or may not be caused by a sexually transmitted disease.

Bacteria

A microscopic one-celled organism.

Yeast infection

Yeast (candida albicans) is a normal inhabitant of the vagina; however, overgrowth of this organism in the vagina may cause vaginal itching and a "cottage cheese"-like discharge. It is not a sexually transmitted disease.

Table 1 The Normal Vulva

What is it?

The vulva is the female external genital organ. It is the area bounded by a fatty pad covered by hair (the mons), the groins, and the back passage (anus). It has outer lips (labia) that cover the clitoris, the inner lips, and the vaginal opening. The tissue around the vaginal opening is called the vestibule.

People use many different names to describe this part of the body. Because women's genitals, unlike men's, are hidden, they can seem mysterious and confusing. It is a good idea to get to know your own body, including your vulva, to help to get rid of this mystery. It is also important to learn correct names for our genitalia so that we can communicate with each other and with our health care provider about our experiences, be they experiences of pleasure or pain.

How do we know what is normal?

Don't be shy! Many women get to know their bodies by taking a good look at their vulvas. This can be done by standing or squatting over a mirror and looking at the vulva. Examining the vulva allows a woman to recognize these common parts (see **Figure 1**).

Mons pubis

This is a hair-covered cushion of fat lying over the pubic bone. The amount of hair can vary from person to person, and the hair tends to get thinner as we get older.

Labia

The word *labia* means "lips" in Latin (and a single 'lip' is a 'labium'). The outer labia are two folds of skin and fatty tissue that are covered with pubic hair after puberty and more or less hide the rest of the vulva. They can be large or small, short or long, and even (like breasts) two different sizes. This is all normal and part of what makes each of us unique. They are sexually sensitive and can swell a little when a woman gets sexually aroused. The vulva is responsive to the female hormone estrogen so that it changes in appearance from infancy through puberty to old age; estrogen makes the labia look fatter.

The inner labia are also sensitive and swell when aroused. These are the folds of skin that go from the clitoral hood to below the vagina. The inner labia can vary in color from pink to brownish black depending on the color of a woman's skin. Like nipples, the inner labia can change color as women mature or during pregnancy. Sometimes they stick out from between the outer labia, and they can be wrinkled or smooth. They are thinner because they don't have any fat in them. The labia may have small sebaceous (oil) glands that look like yellow dots or perhaps there may be papillae, which are tiny regular fleshy pink projections on the inner surface. These are variations of normal and are harmless.

Clitoris

The clitoris is located beneath the point where the inner labia meet. The head, or glans, of the clitoris may appear to be smaller than a pea or bigger than a fingertip. Its size varies from person to person, and it can have different levels of sensitivity. The clitoris is like the male penis and becomes erect during sexual stimulation.

Vestibule

This is the inner area of the inner lips around the opening to the vagina. It is normally a moist area, and a number of glands open into this area to produce secretions that can increase when we are aroused. The urethra (connecting the bladder to the outside) also opens into this area just above the opening of the vagina. The hymen in childhood is a thin membrane partially covering the opening to the vagina. In adults, hymen remnants form a ring around the vaginal opening. The sides of the vestibule are visible as Hart's Line on the inside of the inner lips. The line of change from vulvar skin to the smoother transitional skin of the vulva is called Hart's Line.

Used with permission from the International Society for the Study of Vulvovaginal Disease Patient Information Committee, December 2003.

Table 2 Genital Care for Women

What is it?
Genital care means the way in which women keep their genital area healthy. This part of the body (the vulva)* is made up of skin, moist areas and glands. Secretions (moistness) from the vagina keep it clean and healthy and these secretions are normal. These secretions protect the vagina and the skin.

Are there any problems with washing the genitals?
Yes. The skin and moist surfaces of this part of the body are very delicate. It is important not to wash with harsh chemicals that may irritate the area. Washing too often or rubbing too hard when drying can irritate this skin. If you have problems in this area, washing with plain, lukewarm (not hot) water is best. Using soap, shower gels, and some cleansers can make the problems worse. Your health care provider may be able to suggest a soap substitute.

What is the best way of keeping myself "clean"?
Gently separate the outer "lips," and bathe the inner skin with plain water, using your hands only. Gently pat dry the outer skin. Do not use a hair dryer.

What about clothing?
Wear well-fitting clothing and avoid thongs, girdles, tight jeans, and hose. Wash underclothes in a mild detergent and avoid fabric softeners.

What is best to use for my period?
Disposable menstrual pads and tampons can be used. The best ones are natural cotton or hypoallergenic products. Remember to use ones that fit properly, and change them regularly.

What else should I know?
It is not necessary to wash the vulva every day, and it should not be washed more than once a day. Do not wash the vagina. Do not use wipes, deodorants, douches, or other cosmetic and cleansing products. Women with a problem in this area should use only treatments prescribed by their health care provider.

*You can find more information about the vulva on the ISSVD website, ISSVD.org. (Used with permission from the International Society for the Study of Vulvovaginal Disease Patient Information Committee, June 2006.)

3. It looks funny down there. My labia minora are larger than I would like, and they are uneven. Is this normal?

The size, shape, texture, and color of the inner labia can vary considerably among women, and both of the labia minora are rarely identical. **Figure 2** shows normal labia minora. The labia minora may occasionally enlarge with time or after childbirth. Some women may feel that they get in the way during intercourse or even cause discomfort (e.g., getting caught in a bathing suit). Under select

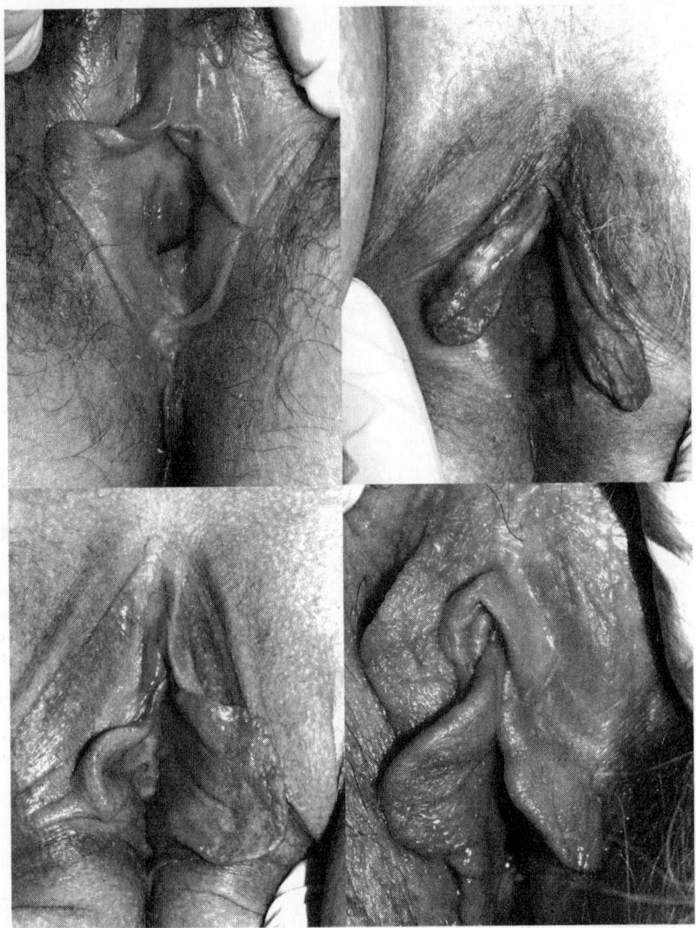

Figure 2 The normal vulva can have a variety of appearances, labia minora are not always symmetrical. (Courtesy of Libby Edwards, MD.)

medical circumstances, they can be made smaller with a procedure called a **labioplasty** or vulvoplasty. This procedure has received a lot of attention recently and is somewhat controversial, as many women are seeking it only for cosmetic reasons. Some health care providers feel that performing this procedure strictly for cosmetic reasons is not appropriate, and the American College of Obstetricians and Gynecologists has also expressed a similar position (ACOG Committee Opinion Number 378, September 2007). Infection, scarring, pain, or changes

Labioplasty

The name for a medical procedure where the labia minora or majora are made smaller. It is sometimes called a vulvoplasty.

in sexual sensation are potential complications of such procedures, which should not be undertaken lightly.

With the influx of immigrants from Africa, a cultural practice known as female circumcision, female cutting, or female genital mutilation is now becoming more widely known. This tradition is practiced in some African countries. Young girls may undergo anything from removal of the clitoral hood, clitoris, excision of the labia minora, and in addition, suturing of the labia majora in the most extensive procedures. These procedures may be performed in less than ideal conditions, and children have died of hemorrhage or infection. The adults may have difficulties with childbirth, urination, recurrent infections, and sexual intercourse. Medical practitioners have been advised to discuss with these participating families the dangers of this practice, hoping that they will not continue it.

Fordyce spots

Yellow-colored sebaceous glands (skin glands) that are visible through the thin labial skin.

Vestibular papillomatosis

More prominent thickening and folding of the skin of the labia and can look like bumps. This is due to the increase in hormone levels that occurs during puberty. Vestibular papillomatosis should not be mistaken for human papilloma virus (genital warts); rather, they are a normal finding.

4. I have little bumps on my labia minora. Does this mean I have warts?

No! Women frequently notice "spots" or bumps. Although sometimes a source of distress, they are actually normal. **Fordyce spots** are merely yellow-colored glands (sebaceous glands) that are visible through the thin (and sensitive!) labial skin. They can enlarge and are more easily seen at puberty, with pregnancy, or hormone use. **Vestibular papillomatosis** is also a normal finding (**Figure 3**). With the increase in hormone levels that occurs during puberty, this can lead to more prominent thickening and folding of the skin of the labia and can look like bumps. Vestibular papillomatosis should not be mistaken for the **human papilloma virus** (HPV) (genital wart) infection, which is discussed later.

Human papilloma virus

The name of the virus that causes genital warts as well as cervical cancer. There are many different strains of this virus. The strains that cause genital warts are different from the ones that are associated with cancer of the cervix.

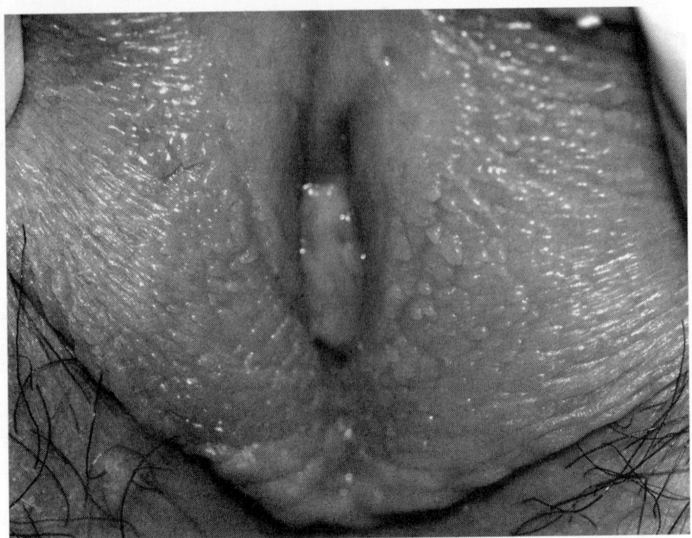

Figure 3 Vestibular papillomatosis. Multiple "bumps" are seen. This is normal and does not represent genital warts. (Courtesy Libby Edwards, MD.)

5. What does it mean when the vagina has an odor?

It is normal for the female genital region to have a mild scent from the secretions and sweat glands. Although there has been much publicity about "feminine hygiene," the slight scent is normal, and more likely than not, it is something your partner is attracted to! An unpleasant vaginal odor can be caused by many things. **Bacterial vaginosis** is one of the most common causes, but other infections, as well as foreign bodies (a retained tampon), poor hygiene, and in very rare circumstances cancer of the **cervix** may be the cause. Bacterial vaginosis (also called "BV") is caused by an overgrowth of certain bacteria that normally live in the vagina after the normal balance of bacteria becomes altered. Women frequently describe a "fishy" odor that is particularly strong after intercourse. Bacterial vaginosis may also be associated with itching, vulvar or vaginal irritation, and a gray-white discharge. It is usually treated with oral or intravaginal antibiotics

Bacterial vaginosis

Caused by an overgrowth of specific bacteria that normally lives in the vagina. Women frequently describe a "fishy" odor that is particularly strong after intercourse. You cannot get bacterial vaginosis from a toilet seat, bed sheets, or swimming pools.

Cervix

A part of internal female anatomy that is the lower part of the uterus (womb).

and is not a **sexually transmitted disease**. A detailed discussion of the types of vaginitis occurs later.

Sexually transmitted disease

Also known as an "STD" or venereal disease, this term refers to any disease transmitted by sexual contact is transmitted via semen, vaginal secretions, or blood during intercourse. Sexually transmitted diseases include HIV, chlamydia, genital herpes, genital warts, gonorrhea, syphilis, and some forms of hepatitis.

Sometimes women forget that they have a tampon in, only to discover it several days later. In such a case, the tampon can result in a vaginal infection and cause a very unpleasant odor. In this case, the tampon should be removed and discarded in a sealed bag, as the odor can permeate the surrounding area. Additionally, if you wear a **pessary** (a plastic or silicone device to support the pelvic organs), you may notice discharge or odor. In this case, the pessary should be removed and cleaned. You should then be evaluated by your health care provider to see whether you should be fitted with a different pessary.

Pessary

A device worn in the vagina to support a displaced uterus, usually made of silicone or plastic.

6. What about waxing and other forms of genital region hair removal?

Although not medically necessary, some women consider hair removal from the genital region necessary for hygiene or aesthetics. It has also been a subject of popular culture, with the "Brazilian wax" touted in magazines as something favored by the famous. In spite of the irritations and infections that can be associated with genital hair removal, gynecologists often find that their patients are quite insistent on continuing the practice. Several methods for temporary genital hair removal include the following: trimming, shaving, using depilatory creams, waxing, sugaring, plucking, and tweezing. All of these methods can be associated with a rash and ingrown hairs. Ingrown hairs can be treated with a mild topical steroid and topical antibiotic, but if infection, rash, or pimples occur, consult your healthcare professional. Also, when the hair grows back, the sharp stubble can cause genital irritation and can rarely become infected. Hair follicles

Folliculitis

Refers to inflammation of hair follicles.

Abscess

A local accumulation of pus that may occur anywhere in the body.

Genital warts

A sexually transmitted disease caused by HPV.

Genital herpes

A sexually transmitted disease caused by herpes simplex virus type 1 or 2, characterized primarily by transient blisters on and around the genitals.

may become infected (also known as **folliculitis**), which is usually a minor infection, but can occasionally develop into significant **abscesses** or soft tissue infections. **Genital warts** and **herpes** can be spread by hair removal methods. More permanent hair removal by laser is also available.

The most common hair removal method is shaving. In order to understand and minimize complications, the following items are advised (see Trager JDK. Pubic hair removal: pearls and pitfalls. *J Pediatr Adolesc Gynecol* 2006;19:117–123):

1. Trim pubic hair first.
2. A warm bath first is helpful.
3. Avoid dry shaving. Use a cream or gel made for the region. Daily application of the product to the skin for a week before use can be used to test for irritation or allergy to the product.
4. Use a new blade each time, and shave in the direction of the hair, gently stretching the skin.
5. Use gentle exfoliation afterward with a loofah. If it is not too irritating, it may help prevent ingrown hairs.
6. Rinse, dry, and use a special pubic aftershave after testing as before for irritation or allergy.
7. Use daily moisturizing and washing.

Depilatory creams specifically formulated for the bikini region are available but can be irritating or provoke allergy, just as other products can in this sensitive area.

Perineum

The area in front of the anus extending to the fourchette of the vulva in the female.

Waxing has become quite popular. Different amounts of hair can be removed, ranging from the hair that would protrude from a bikini below the navel and at the upper thighs to varying shapes ("landing strip," triangle, etc.) to almost or complete hair removal. Brazilian waxes remove hair from the **perineum**, the area between the vagina and anus, as well as the perianal area. In these procedures, warm wax is applied. Then a muslin strip is applied to the warm wax, and the hair is ripped out quickly. This can be quite painful, particularly the first time. Taking ibuprofen before waxing may be helpful. Ingrown hairs and bumps are common, although the results last for several weeks. Serious infections can rarely occur. Sugaring is similar to waxing, with a sugar paste used instead. If waxing is chosen as a hair removal method, make sure that you use a trained aesthetician.

7. *What about body jewelry in the genital region?*

Genital piercing is practiced as a form of self-expression. Some individuals report increased sexual satisfaction, although the evidence for this is unverified. Piercing of the labia majora, minora, or the hood of the clitoris has become more common, although not widespread. Descriptions of variety of different piercing sites can be found on the Internet. Occasionally, piercing through the body of the clitoris is performed but is not without some risks of bleeding and/or infection. Healing varies by site but can be weeks to months. Other potential complications can include allergic reactions, difficulties with hygiene, scarring, trauma to the partner's genitalia, swallowing/choking on loose jewelry, or injury to teeth. Body jewelry should be removed before childbirth.

Genital piercing should be performed by a trained individual. Make sure that a sterile technique is used.

Genital piercing should be performed by a trained individual. Make sure that a sterile technique is used. The individual doing the piercing should wash his or her hands and use sterile gloves. Needles used should be disposable. Anything nondisposable should be sterilized in an autoclave. Scrupulous attention to aftercare to avoid infection is also necessary.

PART TWO

Vulvar Pain

What could cause pain in the vulva?

Intercourse has become painful for me.
What could be the problem?

Sometimes the opening to my vagina splits open,
causing a lot of pain with intercourse.
Why does this happen?

More . . .

8. *What could cause pain in the vulva?*

A multitude of conditions can cause vulvar pain. Some of the more common causes include infections such as with yeast or herpes. Most of the sexually transmitted diseases, such as **syphilis**, that cause ulcers are painless, but **chancroid**, a rare sexually transmitted disease in the United States, can cause a painful ulcer. Occasionally, genital warts can cause pain, especially if they become infected. Atrophy caused by a loss of female hormones (such as after going through menopause) can cause vulvar pain because the tissues become thin and therefore more sensitive. A condition called **vulvodynia** is a vulvar pain syndrome in which the cause is unknown. The localized form has previously been called vulvar vestibulitis syndrome. It can make intercourse painful or impossible and can interfere with other daily activities, such as tampon use, wearing of certain clothing, bicycle riding, and so forth. Any type of touch may be painful. A more generalized form of vulvodynia may hurt, even without touch. It is important to see a healthcare provider who is familiar with these conditions because there may be nothing visible to the naked eye on examination. A variety of treatments, including medication, and physical therapy can be helpful. Patients with this condition can find useful information at *http://www.nva.org* and *htpp://www.issvd.org.*

Skin disorders that affect the vulva can also cause discomfort. These include **lichen sclerosus, lichen planus**, and **plasma cell (Zoon's) vulvitis**, a very rare condition. In women who have **lichen simplex chronicus** and scratch frequently, the skin can become irritated and infected, thus causing pain. Other causes of pain include spasms of the muscles of the pelvic floor (called levator ani spasm or pelvic floor dysfunction), which can

Syphilis

A specific sexually transmitted disease which can be associated with a rash in early stages and with neurological impairment in late stages of the disease. In most cases, syphilis can be treated with penicillin.

Chancroid

A soft, highly infectious, nonsyphilitic venereal ulcer of the genital region, caused by the bacillus *Hemophilus ducreyi.*

Vulvodynia

Term used for a vulvar pain syndrome, in which the cause is unknown.

Lichen sclerosus

A dermatologic disorder that may affect the vulva. The vulvar skin becomes thin or atrophic, white, and wrinkly, associated with severe itching.

Lichen planus

A rare inflammatory, noninfectious, noncontagious skin disorder that may be found in many areas of the body, including the genitalia and mouth.

cause "referred" pain to the vulvar area. Some have proposed that high levels of **oxalate crystals** in the urine can cause vulvar pain. Allergic reactions or environmental irritants such as soaps, detergents, douches, and sprays can cause vulvar discomfort as well.

9. Intercourse has become painful for me. What could be the problem?

Dyspareunia (pronounced "dis-par-une-ee-ah"), the medical term for painful sexual intercourse, is a common complaint among women of all ages. Many women report occasional pain with intercourse, but some women have pain each time they attempt to have sexual relations. This can be upsetting to the woman and can cause strain in her relationship with her partner. The pain with intercourse can occur "on entry," meaning that there is pain as soon as something touches the labia minora or vaginal opening, or the pain can be inside, known as "deep" dyspareunia. Fortunately, the cause of the pain can usually be identified and treated. Perhaps one of the most common conditions associated with painful intercourse is inadequate lubrication (e.g., because of a lack of estrogen or foreplay), which may cause generalized discomfort (for both partners). A lack of lubrication may require the addition of hormones in the postmenopausal woman. Adequate foreplay is also important, and specific water-based lubricants may be helpful. Oil-based lubricants such as mineral oil or petroleum jelly may lessen the effectiveness of latex condoms for both sexually transmitted disease and pregnancy prevention.

Pain immediately on penetration can be caused by infections, which can cause irritation of the vulvar and vaginal tissues, such as with yeast or bacterial vaginosis.

Lichen simplex chronicus

Also called squamous cell hyperlasia; lichen simplex chronicus is a thickening of the vulvar skin that is the result of an uninterrupted cycle of itching and scratching. The more one itches, the more one scratches, which in turn induces more itching.

Plasma cell vulvitis

Also known as Zoon's vulvitis, this is a rare dermatologic condition that can affect the vulva.

Oxalate crystal

Oxalate crystals are normal in urine, but in high amounts may contribute to vulvar pain, although this hasn't been established with certainty.

Dyspareunia

The medical term for painful sexual intercourse. There are many causes of dyspareunia, and it is a common complaint among women of all ages.

Anything that causes a break in the skin of the vulva or vagina such as a herpes blister, a scrape, or a fissure (see Question 10) can cause intense pain with intercourse. **Vestibulodynia**, or pain specifically in the vulvar vestibule, can cause entrance dyspareunia and may be primary or secondary (see earlier questions). Occasionally, women may have a **hymen** that remains partially intact even after several attempts at intercourse; this can cause pain with future attempts at penetration. Finally, dermatologic conditions such as lichen sclerosus and lichen planus, which may damage the vulvar skin and make it tender, can cause painful penetration. The treatment of entrance dyspareunia depends on the cause.

Vestibulodynia

Pain specifically in the vulvar vestibule.

Hymen

A fold of mucous membrane partly closing the external orifice of the vagina.

Ovarian cysts

Fluid fulled growths in the ovary, which may be related to ovulation, or may reflect a benign or rarely malignant new growth.

Pelvic organ prolapse

Protrusion or descent of any of the female pelvic organs such as the uterus, vagina, bladder, or rectum.

Leiomyoma

Benign tumors of the uterus, also known as "fibroids."

Endometriosis

The presence of endometrial tissue in an incorrect location. In some women, it is associated with pain and infertility. Rarely, it occurs on the vulva.

Deep dyspareunia occurs when deep penile penetration causes pain and may vary with the position used during intercourse. Several conditions are associated with deep dyspareunia, including levator ani muscle spasm, which is an involuntary spasm of the pelvic muscles, **ovarian cysts** (which may rupture, leading to further discomfort), severe constipation, **pelvic organ prolapse** (descent of the uterus, bladder, and vagina), intrapelvic adhesions (caused by scar tissue from prior surgery or an infection), large **leiomyoma** (also called fibroids, which are benign growths of the uterus), and **endometriosis**. The diagnosis and treatment of the causes of entrance or deep dyspareunia may require several office visits to your gynecologist or other medical specialists and sometimes imaging or other studies.

Pain can occasionally occur after intercourse. This can be due to uterine contractions with orgasm, or rarely, the woman may have an allergy to her partner's sperm in which she experiences burning and redness in the vagina and the vulva.

10. Sometimes the opening to my vagina splits open, causing a lot of pain with intercourse. Why does this happen?

This is known as **granuloma fissuratum**. It is characterized by recurrent splitting of the tissue at the 6-o'clock position of the vestibule, the posterior fourchette, and severe pain with intercourse, tampon insertion, or vaginal examination. No one is sure why this occurs, although there may be several explanations. Sometimes it can occur at the site of a prior repair (**episiotomy**) or tear from childbirth. Fortunately, most cases of granuloma fissuratum may be successfully treated medically or surgically.

Granuloma fissuratum

Refers to splitting or "fissuring" of the female vulva.

Episiotomy

Refers to a surgical incision of the perineum to enlarge the vagina and so facilitate delivery during childbirth.

PART THREE

Vaginal Discharge and Itching

What is considered normal vaginal discharge?

What causes vulvar itching?

Is it okay to be sexually active while being treated for vaginal discharge?

More . . .

11. What is considered normal vaginal discharge?

All women experience some vaginal discharge or moisture. This helps the vagina stay healthy by regularly flushing it and maintaining a healthy pH (acid base balance). Most women have some vaginal discharge that varies throughout their menstrual cycle. Even very young women who have not begun menstruating can have vaginal discharge. It is common to notice some discharge after using the bathroom or to find wet or dried discharge on your underwear. Normal vaginal discharge can change throughout the menstrual cycle, becoming a bit thicker during mid cycle when you are ovulating. Normal vaginal discharge is usually white or clear and odorless or has a very mild odor.

Most women have some vaginal discharge that varies throughout their menstrual cycle.

Signs that that there may be a problem include an increase in the amount of discharge, a change in the smell or the color of the discharge, and vulvar or vaginal irritation or burning.

An abnormal vaginal discharge would be an increase in the amount that you usually experience, as well as a yellow or green color with a fishy or foul odor. A change in the texture from pasty or sticky (normal) to a clumpy, "cottage cheese"-like discharge is also abnormal.

If you feel that you have abnormal vaginal discharge, see your health care provider, ideally on a day when you feel that your discharge is abnormal. It is better to be seen before you treat yourself with an over-the-counter medication so that your provider can appropriately evaluate you. Not all discharges are yeast infections!

12. What is abnormal vaginal discharge? Does it mean that I have cancer or a sexually transmitted disease?

The glands inside the vagina and cervix make small amounts of fluid that may come out of the vagina; this is normal and is known as "**physiologic discharge**." This normal discharge helps to keep the vagina healthy and clean. It is usually clear or white and thin and is typically odorless. Some women experience a thicker (like egg whites) discharge during the middle of their menstrual cycle. This is associated with ovulation (when an ovary releases an egg). The discharge may also be thicker while you are nursing or during sexual arousal. Thus, some vaginal discharge is normal and does not necessarily mean that you have a sexually transmitted disease or cancer.

Physiologic discharge

Normal vaginal discharge caused by the glands inside the vagina and cervix that make small amounts of fluid that may come out of the vagina. This normal discharge helps to keep the vaginal healthy and clean.

Trichomonas

A sexually transmitted disease caused by a parasite, Trichomonas vaginalis. It often presents with a thin, watery vaginal discharge and itching.

Signs that there may be a problem include an increase in the amount of discharge, a change in the smell or the color of the discharge, and vulvar or vaginal irritation or burning. Discharge that is stained with blood (if not during your period) is also abnormal.

Gonorrhea

A sexually transmitted disease which may be asymptomatic in women or may cause yellow or green vaginal discharge. It is treated with antibiotics.

Sexually transmitted diseases are a common cause of abnormal vaginal discharge. **Trichomonas** may cause a thin, watery, green or grayish discharge. **Gonorrhea** and **chlamydia** can be associated with a thick, yellow-green discharge. Genital herpes, which causes superficial ulcers on the vulva and or vagina, can bleed a bit, making the discharge red, or blood tinged. Bacterial vaginosis may also cause an abnormal discharge that is often grey and bubbly. Some women notice a particularly strong and fishy odor after intercourse. A yeast infection can cause a thick, "cottage cheese"-like discharge. It is uncommon for a female malignancy to present with vaginal discharge, but it can. Signs of a possible malignancy include watery or bloody discharge.

Chlamydia

A sexually transmitted disease that may be asymptomatic in women or may cause yellow or green vaginal discharge. Chlamydia, like gonorrhea, may be associated with pelvic inflammatory disease and infertility.

13. What should I do about discharge?

Treatment of the discharge is dependent on the cause. If you feel that your discharge is not normal (as described previously here), you should be evaluated by your health care provider. Self-treatment is usually not best. Tests that might be performed include a **wet mount**, which involves looking at a sample of the discharge in salt water under the microscope. Other tests include a **KOH prep**, which is where a sample of the discharge is put in a potassium hydrochloride solution and examined under the microscope. A KOH (potassium hydroxide) prep is used to diagnose a yeast infection. It may also release the characteristic fishy odor associated with bacterial vaginosis. This is called a "whiff" test. Your provider may also culture the vagina with a cotton swab and send it to the laboratory. The results usually take a few days to come back. After your health care provider has made the diagnosis, he or she will be able to recommend appropriate treatment. Treatment may be given based on clinical impression as well, but if the problem does not clear up, additional testing may be needed.

Wet mount

Term for a test where a few drops of saline and vaginal discharge are applied to a slide and examined under a microscope.

KOH prep

"KOH" is the chemical name for "potassium hydroxide," which is mixed with a small sample of vaginal discharge and examined under a microscope to diagnose a yeast infection.

If you feel that your discharge is not normal (as described previously here), you should be evaluated by your health care provider. Self-treatment is usually not best.

14. What is vaginitis?

The term "itis" means inflammation; therefore, vaginitis means inflammation of the vagina. Vaginitis is frequently caused by a change in the balance of the normal bacteria that live in the vagina (such as bacterial vaginosis or yeast) or by an infection with an organism that is not normally part of the vaginal flora (such as trichomonas). After women have gone through menopause and have lower levels of estrogen, they may get atrophic vaginitis, a specific type of vaginitis. Vaginitis typically presents with discharge, itching, rawness or pain, and discomfort with intercourse. The treatment of vaginitis depends on which type you have. Women commonly self-treat and often assume that a vaginal discharge is a yeast infection, but this is frequently the wrong diagnosis! If vaginitis does not clear up after use of an over-the-counter yeast medication or seems atypical in any way, evaluation by a healthcare practitioner should be sought. Douching is not advisable, as it may make the condition worse and may actually lead to worse inflammatory problems (see Question 2).

15. What is a yeast infection?

A yeast infection, also known as **candidiasis**, is not really an infection. Yeast (*Candida albicans*) is a normal inhabitant of the vagina; however, if it overgrows and overtakes the other healthy organisms in the vagina, you may have vaginal itching, a characteristic white, "cottage cheese"-like discharge, redness, swelling or itching around the vulva, and pain or burning during intercourse and are said to have a "yeast infection" of the vagina. It is *not* a sexually transmitted disease. The most common organism is *C. albicans*, but it may be caused by other yeast organisms. Yeast infections usually occur in moist areas of the body such as in the mouth, where it is called "thrush," and moist areas of the skin. Factors that may cause a yeast infection include hormonal changes with the menstrual cycle (some women notice that they get a yeast infection right before their period) and conditions that may affect the immune system and lead to candida overgrowth such as pregnancy and stress. Some medications are associated with yeast infections such as oral contraceptive pills and steroids. Antibiotics sometimes kill the good, as well as the bad, bacteria that keep your vagina healthy, thus allowing an overgrowth of yeast. If you are prone to yeast infections, using a medication for

Candidiasis

Any of a variety of infections caused by fungi of the genus *Candida*, occurring most often in the mouth, respiratory tract, or vagina.

Overgrowth of yeast (Candida albicans) may cause vaginal itching, a characteristic white, "cottage cheese"-like discharge, redness, swelling or itching around the vulva, and pain or burning during intercourse.

yeast at the same time as you are taking the antibiotics may sometimes ward off a yeast infection. Wearing thong underwear may predispose you to a yeast infection because Candida species that normally live in the colon can more easily reach the vagina, tracking along the thong. Tight clothing can trap heat and moisture, creating an ideal environment for yeast to thrive. Loose cotton underwear is better for preventing this. Finally, women with poorly controlled diabetes who have elevated blood glucose levels may get yeast infections more often.

16. What else could cause vaginal discharge?

If your discharge is not due to the normal vaginal secretions and not due to a sexually transmitted disease, a yeast infection, or other common causes of vaginitis such as trichomonas or bacterial vaginosis, it may be due to a maligancy, a very rare case of vaginal discharge. Another uncommon cause is a poorly understood condition called **desquamative inflammatory vaginitis**. Desquamative inflammatory vaginitis is characterized by copious, yellow-green discharge. It is unclear whether it is associated with lichen planus or what its causes are. It is more common in postmenopausal women. Some women have reported that the discharge of desquamative inflammatory vaginitis is so sticky that is doesn't come out of their underwear, even after washing it in hot water. Women with this condition commonly report vulvar irritation caused by the sticky discharge coating the vulva.

Desquamative inflammatory vaginitis

A specific type of vaginitis that is characterized by copious, yellow-green discharge. It is not associated with a specific infecting organism.

There is no clear consensus for how to diagnose desquamative inflammatory vaginitis. Typically is it diagnosed by patient history, physical examination, and a wet prep (saline solution) of the discharge; however, desquamative inflammatory vaginitis is treatable, typically with a combination of vaginal antibiotics, low-potency steroids, and topical estrogen.

17. What causes vulvar itching?

Many things can cause vulvar itching, including a variety of skin conditions such as lichen sclerosus, lichen simplex chronicus, and genital warts. Other causes include vaginitis due to as bacterial vaginosis or **trichomoniasis**. The vaginal discharge from these conditions may irritate the vulva, causing itching. Rarely, a malignancy can cause vulvar itching. If you have recurrent vulvar itching, you should be evaluated by a health care provider who is knowledgeable about vulvar disease. Itching may also reflect irritation or allergy from a variety of products you may be using on your genital region or irritation from tight clothing.

If you have recurrent vulvar itching, you should be evaluated by a health care provider who is knowledgeable about vulvar disease.

Melinda's comments:

I had vulvar itching for weeks but was too embarrassed to tell my doctor. I stopped having relations with my boyfriend. As it turned out, I had bacterial vaginosis, which was easily treated with vaginal antibiotics. I started to feel better within a few days. I was symptom free after a week, and I felt as if I had my life back!

Trichomoniasis
A form of vagintis caused by Trichomoniasis vaginalis, it can cause a yellow-green bubble discharge.

Vulvar cancer
The fourth most common female genital tract cancer and comprises 5% of malignancies of the female genital tract. Squamous cell carcinoma is the most common type of vulvar cancer.

18. How is vulvar itching treated?

The treatment for vulvar itching depends on the cause. Infections may require oral or topical treatment with antibiotics. Sometimes an early **vulvar cancer**, even before it can be seen, can cause itching. These early cancers can be removed in a variety of ways. A gynecologist or dermatologist who is experienced in vulvar diseases should evaluate skin conditions such as lichen sclerosus and lichen simplex chronicus. These conditions are often diagnosed with a **biopsy** of the itchy area and are usually readily treated with medications. If an infection is suspected as the cause of the itching, a culture is frequently performed so that the exact bacteria, fungus, or virus causing the infection can be identified. Treatment (such as with an antibiotic or a steroid) is then based on these findings. Vulvar itching often responds to cold ice packs, which can provide temporary relief but will not solve the underlying problem. Some conditions may require topical steroids that are prescribed by a healthcare provider. Over-the-counter itch creams containing benzocaine can cause significant dermatitis and cause marked worsening of the irritation and itching. These should be avoided. Sometimes women may scratch in their sleep. In this case, an oral medication that decreases the itching may provide some relief while the underlying problem is being treated. Patients must stop scratching in order to treat the condition.

Biopsy

A small piece of tissue is removed, usually performed in the office with local anesthesia so that a diagnosis can be made.

19. What is bacterial vaginosis?

Bacterial vaginosis is the most common vaginal infection in women of childbearing age. It actually is not an infection but is an overgrowth of a mixture of bacteria that normally inhabit the vagina so that they overtake the bacteria that provide a healthy vaginal environment. A healthy vaginal environment contains "good" bacteria called **lactobacilli** (and a few other types). Lactobacilli maintain a healthy acidic environment in the vagina, thus inhibiting the growth of "harmful" bacteria. When the acidity in the vagina is altered, the normal balance of bacteria in the vagina may change so that there is an

Lactobacilli

A special type of bacteria normally found in the vagina. They maintain a healthy acidic environment in the vagina that inhibits the growth of other "harmful" bacteria and keeps the vagina healthy.

overgrowth of bacteria that can cause problems in large numbers. Although the exact cause of bacterial vaginosis is unknown, the overgrowth of harmful bacteria may contribute to the development of bacterial vaginosis. You cannot get bacterial vaginosis from toilet seats, bed sheets, or swimming pools.

Although any woman can get bacterial vaginosis and it is not a sexually transmitted disease, certain behaviors can upset the normal balance of bacteria in the vagina, thereby putting a woman at increased risk of getting bacterial vaginosis. These include having a new sexual partner or multiple partners, douching, and the use of an intrauterine device for contraception.

Although the exact cause of bacterial vaginosis is unknown, the overgrowth of harmful bacteria may contribute to the development of bacterial vaginosis.

20. How is bacterial vaginosis diagnosed?

Signs of bacterial vaginosis can include an abnormal grey frothy vaginal discharge, an unpleasant odor, especially after intercourse (some women report a strong fishy odor), pain, and itching or burning on the outside of the vagina. Bacterial vaginosis is diagnosed by a health care provider, usually by looking at vaginal secretions under the microscope. A "whiff" test consists of adding a few drops of potassium hydroxide to the vaginal secretions on the slide. This alters the pH from acidic to basic and reproduces the characteristic "fishy" odor. Wet smears can show "clue cells," which are normal vaginal cells coated with the bacteria causing the condition and are diagnostic of bacterial vaginosis. Clue cells can also be seen on **Pap smears** but may not be associated with clinical symptoms of bacterial vaginosis.

Pap smear

Short for "Papanicolaou" test, named after the physician who described taking a sample of cells from a woman's cervix as a way to screen for cervical cancer.

21. What are the complications of having bacterial vaginosis?

Usually there are no complications from having bacterial vaginosis, except that it can be unpleasant.

Usually there are no complications from having bacterial vaginosis, except that it can be unpleasant. If you are pregnant, however, bacterial vaginosis may increase your risk of preterm labor, although testing and treating for bacterial vaginosis in pregnancy are controversial. Bacterial vaginosis has been associated with an increased risk of developing an infection after a procedure such as a hysterectomy or a dilation and curettage (D&C). Having bacterial vaginosis can increase a woman's susceptibility to infection with HIV as well as other sexually transmitted infections if exposed.

22. How is bacterial vaginosis treated?

Sometimes bacterial vaginosis will resolve without any treatment at all; however, all women with symptoms associated with bacterial vaginosis should be treated. Men generally do not need to be treated. Bacterial vaginosis is treated with prescription antibiotics such as metronidazole or clindamycin. Bacterial vaginosis may recur after treatment.

23. Is it okay to be sexually active while being treated for vaginal discharge?

Generally speaking, this is not a good idea. If you are being treated for a sexually transmitted disease, your chance of getting the infection again increases, especially if your partner has not been evaluated and treated if necessary. If you are being treated for a yeast infection with a cream, for example, the medication may not be as effective, and you would risk being incompletely treated. Also, if the cause of your discharge is causing pain, be sure you are completely treated and pain free before engaging in something such as sexual activity, as this could make the pain worse.

24. How do I prevent vaginitis?

You can help prevent vaginitis by doing the following:

1. Wipe from the front to the back after using the toilet. This can help to prevent bacteria from the anal area from getting into the vagina.
2. Wear cotton underwear during the day and no underwear at night. Cotton is a natural fiber that will allow air to reach your skin better than a synthetic fabric. The vulvar area needs to "breathe."
3. Avoid wearing tight pants and pantyhose for long periods of time.
4. Refrain from staying in a wet bathing suit.
5. Do not douche. A normal vagina is self-cleaning. If there is a problem with discharge or odor, this needs to be evaluated. Douching can make things worse and may increase the chance of pelvic inflammatory disease as well.

PART FOUR

Sexually Transmitted Diseases

When am I contagious, and how can transmission be prevented?

Will having genital warts affect my fertility?

What is the HPV vaccine?

More . . .

25. I have herpes. What does that mean?

Genital herpes is very common, affecting about 20% to 25% of adults in the United States. Genital herpes is caused by the **Herpes simplex virus** type 1 or type 2 (HSV-1 and HSV-2), which are typically transmitted through sexual contact. Although HSV-1 is more commonly associated with cold sores around the mouth and HSV-2 is more commonly associated with genital herpes, either type can cause herpes outbreaks in either location. Signs of infection include a blister(s) in the genital area, as well as redness, itching, and/or pain. Some women get "prodromal" symptoms, which include discomfort or itchiness in the area before a visible lesion appears. After the blister breaks, it leaves a sensitive, sometimes painful sore (or "ulcer") that can take a few weeks to heal. Sometimes active infection is more subtle, with the person noting only a tingling sensation. People are sometimes really upset when they find out that they have genital herpes, and it can be associated with a lot of emotional distress. Herpes is a very common condition, however, and if you have it, you should not blame yourself. One person of four on the bus with you probably also has it! Although the first infection (also known as the primary outbreak) can be very unpleasant, recurrences (recurrent outbreaks) are often minor in terms of physical symptoms. Recurrent outbreaks may occur as often as once a month (uncommon) or every few years. Be sure to discuss herpes with your provider, especially if you are pregnant, as herpes is dangerous for the newborn and precautions, such as a possible cesarean delivery, can be taken.

Herpes simplex virus

The name of the virus that causes genital herpes.

Although HSV-1 is more commonly associated with cold sores around the mouth and HSV-2 is more commonly associated with genital herpes, either type can cause herpes outbreaks in either location.

26. How do I know if I have herpes?

Herpes infections can be "primary," the name for a first-time infection, or "recurrent." The primary infection refers to the first time you have an episode, which usually occurs within 2 weeks after the virus is transmitted. Women experience tingling and pain that is sometimes accompanied by a fever, swollen glands, particularly in the groin, and a general sense of not feeling well or having the "flu." These symptoms are usually accompanied by multiple blisters. When they break, urination may be extremely painful, as the urine hits the open ulcers, and rarely, patients end up in the emergency room because of the pain on urination. Subsequent outbreaks are usually much less painful. Sometimes women don't get a blister and may only have mild itching or discomfort. The diagnosis of herpes can be made by visual inspection if the infection presents as the typical ulcer; however, a definitive diagnosis is made when your health care provider takes a culture or smear of the blister/ulcer. Blood tests are sometimes helpful as well. Typically, the first infection or "outbreak" is usually the most uncomfortable. Recurrent infections occur at variable intervals after the primary infection and can occur a month to years later. The number of outbreaks usually decreases with time. Medication (**suppression therapy**) is available to decrease the frequency of outbreaks.

Suppression therapy

Therapy to prevent or decrease the number of outbreaks.

Beth's comments:

After I had been with my boyfriend for 4 years, I developed painful blisters in the genital region. The pain was almost unbearable, and I had difficulty urinating. I had no idea what was happening to me, and I went to my gynecologist who diagnosed me with genital herpes. Up until that point, I had never thought about sexually transmitted diseases—they were always something that happened to other people. I was devastated not only that I had herpes but that my long-term boyfriend had cheated on me.

My doctor gave me antiviral medication that I took by mouth and applied to the blisters. The medication began to work pretty quickly, and I began to feel better. The blisters popped on their own and turned into sores that were completely gone about 2 weeks later. That was 2 years ago; I have had one more outbreak since then, which occurred when I was stressed out while studying for final exams.

Although this was a hurtful experience for me, I have come to accept the fact that I carry herpes. On a day-to-day basis, it is not something that I even think about. When I felt tingling and burning before the blisters appeared during the second episode, I knew what to do, and I started medication right away. The second episode was much shorter than the first!

I have a new boyfriend now, and when I told him my story, he was fine with it. He thanked me for my honesty, and we have an active sexual relationship and always use condoms.

27. Does genital herpes cause cancer?

Genital herpes has not been shown to cause cancer. In fact, serious complications are rarely associated with genital herpes, although anxiety occurs in those who know that they are infected. However, genital herpes can be serious if you are pregnant and are about to deliver because there is a chance that you could pass the infection to the baby; therefore, women with active genital herpes are usually offered a cesarean delivery at the time of delivery (as long as their bag of water is not ruptured for a long time). If you are pregnant and know or suspect that you have herpes, notify your health care provider. You should discuss a plan for notifying your provider when you either break your water or go into labor.

Genital herpes can be serious if you are pregnant and are about to deliver because there is a chance that you could pass the infection to the baby; therefore, women with active genital herpes are usually offered a cesarean delivery at the time of delivery (as long as their bag of water isn't ruptured for a long time).

28. When am I contagious, and how can transmission be prevented?

Anytime you have a visible infection, either a blister or a healing ulcer, you are contagious. Also, if you have "prodromal" symptoms such as tingling, discomfort, and itchiness, you may be contagious, even though nothing may be visible on the skin. You may also be contagious when you have no symptoms at all. Women are more likely to become infected with herpes than men.

Herpes may also increase the spread of other sexually transmitted diseases, especially HIV, probably because herpes breaks the protective barrier of the skin, allowing the HIV to get in.

The best way to prevent transmission is to refrain from sexual contact if one of the partners has prodromal symptoms or an active lesion. Barrier methods such as condoms can greatly reduce transmission but will not eliminate the risk. Suppressive medication can also help but cannot totally eliminate transmission.

29. How is genital herpes treated?

After you have herpes, you never "get rid" of the virus; instead, it stays dormant in the nerves and can recur at any time, especially under times of stress. This is similar to other viruses, such as the virus that causes chicken pox (a virus in the same family as herpes, by the way),

Although there is no treatment that can cure herpes, antiviral medications can shorten the duration of an outbreak and decrease the associated discomfort.

which stays in the system and can show up years later as shingles. Although there is no treatment that can cure herpes, antiviral medications can shorten the duration of an outbreak and decrease the associated discomfort. For people who suffer from frequent outbreaks, suppression therapy can decrease the frequency and severity of outbreaks. Finally, suppressive therapy can decrease transmission to a sexual partner.

30. What is trichomonas?

Trichomonas vaginalis is a microscopic parasite. Infection with this organism is called trichomoniasis or a "trich infection." It is one of the most common sexually transmitted diseases, mainly affecting sexually active women. In North America (the organism is found worldwide), there are an estimated 8 million cases a year.

Trichomoniasis is spread through sexual activity and cannot be obtained from a toilet seat. Men usually do not have symptoms (asymptomatic) and therefore are unaware that they are infected and capable of spreading the infection. Women may be asymptomatic—trichomonas may be seen on a Pap smear, or some women may have a foul-smelling, frothy yellow-green vaginal discharge, vaginal itching, vaginal redness, pain during sexual intercourse, and the urge to urinate.

31. How is trichomoniasis diagnosed?

Your health care provider will perform a pelvic examination (usually a speculum is placed into the vagina) to collect a sample of vaginal secretions. The secretions are then examined under the microscope where the parasite can be seen. Culturing the secretions for the parasite is actually the best way to diagnose the infection, but results can take up to a week. As no test is 100% accurate, your health care provider may perform more than one test for diagnosis. Occasionally, women will complain of symptoms of a urinary tract infection, and trichomoniasis is found to be the cause. Although trichomonas can be identified on a Pap smear, a Pap smear is not very sensitive for detecting trichomonas and will miss many cases; therefore, although the information is useful, the Pap is not considered for a method to diagnose trichomonas.

If you think you may have vaginal trichomoniasis, you and your partner should see a health care provider. Both partners should be diagnosed and treated; otherwise, the partner who is not treated may reinfect the other. After you are infected and have been treated, this does not mean that you are immune to trichomonas. It is possible to become reinfected. Finally, if you know that you have one sexually transmitted disease, you may have others because of your increased exposure risk. Discuss with your health care provider the possibility of performing a "sexually transmitted disease panel," which tests for many other types of infections.

32. How is trichomoniasis treated? How is it prevented?

Trichomoniasis is almost always treated with a course of oral antibiotics that is specific for the organism. Occasionally vaginal medication is used. The most common oral medication is metronidazole, which has been shown to be highly effective and well tolerated. Some patients do experience nausea or stomach upset. You should not drink any alcohol while taking metronidazole, as it can lead to nausea and vomiting.

Trichomoniasis is almost always treated with a course of oral antibiotics that is specific for the organism. Occasionally vaginal medication is used.

The best way to prevent trichomoniasis, as with all sexually transmitted diseases, is with abstinence. Limiting the number of sexual partners will also decrease your risk of contracting a sexually transmitted disease. Alternatively, a latex condom should be used if you have sexual intercourse. Natural lambskin condoms are not as effective at preventing the transmission of sexually transmitted diseases. Finally, although oral contraceptive pills, diaphragms, sponges, injectable medications, and spermicides may be effective means of contraception, they do not necessarily prevent sexually transmitted diseases. Having trichomonas may increase the risk of acquiring HIV if exposed to it sexually.

33. I was told that I have genital warts. What does this mean?

Genital warts are caused by HPV, which is transmitted via sexual contact. Over 30 types of HPV can be sexually transmitted, and they affect the genital area in both men and women. They may not show up at all or may appear as "warts" on the skin of the vulva, vagina, anus, penis, and rectum. About 20 million people in the Unites States have HPV, and by age 50, about 80% of sexually active women will have acquired genital HPV. Most, however, will not have visible genital warts. The warts on other parts of the skin or soles of the feet (plantar warts) are caused by different HPV types than the ones that affect the genital region.

Beth's comments:

Although genital warts may be treated in a number of ways, the body never completely eradicates HPV. This can be frustrating and a bit nerve racking—you may start to wonder whether another one is going to pop up, and there is no sure way to guarantee that one won't pop up again. On the other hand, you may never see a wart again for the rest of your life. Although we can't predict if and when another wart will appear, there is comfort in knowing that there are several safe treatments for genital warts. It is also important to bear in mind that the same types of HPV that cause genital warts do not usually cause cervical cancer.

34. How are genital warts diagnosed?

Genital warts might be diagnosed based on their appearance. Most HPV infections are asymptomatic, especially in men, who may have no visible lumps or bumps because the warts may be in their urethra. Frequently, there are no signs or symptoms, and most people don't know that they are infected. Some people get a visible wart that is variable in appearance; it can be soft, pink, raised or flat, single or in groups, and small or large.

Frequently, there are no signs or symptoms of genital warts, and most people don't know that they are infected.

Although there is a specific test that can identify HPV in cervical swabs, women are increasingly being diagnosed with cervical or vaginal HPV because they have had an abnormal Pap smear or are screened for cervical HPV at the time of their Pap smear if they are over 30 years old. Because HPV is so common and usually cleared to the point of indetectability on a screening test by itself, testing younger women for HPV routinely would result in unnecessary treatments for some who are not destined to develop serious lesions (precancers). Of course, this varies with the individual patient and should be discussed with your provider. A Pap smear is a screening test for cervical cancer. Almost all cases of cervical cancer are related to HPV infection (Question 39).

35. Will having genital warts affect my fertility?

Genital warts have not been shown to reduce fertility; however, having a sexually transmitted infection means that you are at increased risk for other sexually transmitted infections, via the same sexual exposures, and some of them, like gonorrhea or chlamydia, can affect your fertility.

36. Did I get genital warts from my partner?

It is possible. Don't break up with them yet, however! After sexual contact with an infected partner, a wart may appear within weeks or months, or not at all. HPV can remain dormant in your system and appear months or years later, unrelated to any current sexual exposure. Some people who carry HPV *never* notice a wart. The exact latency period is unknown; therefore, if you have discovered a wart, you may not have contracted HPV from your current partner. Also, reassure your partner that it doesn't mean that you have had other recent contacts as well, if that is the case.

Because most HPV is sexually transmitted, you likely got it from a sexual partner. Rarely, it is thought that HPV can be caught from hand to genital contact, or theoretically, towels (not toilet seats!), although most sexually transmitted organisms do not live long on inanimate objects. It is unclear, however, how long HPV can stay in the system without showing signs; thus, it can be from a sexual encounter that took place a long time ago. It should not be taken as a sign that one's current partner has been unfaithful. HPV is extremely common, and it is estimated that over 75% of sexually active people will contract HPV over their lifetimes; therefore, anyone who is sexually active may contract HPV. The immune system is geared to clear the virus, and thus, most people remove it from their system without ever knowing they have had it; however, the persistence of the virus is a risk factor for cancers that are associated with certain high-risk types of HPV (not all types!).

The types of HPV that lead to visible warts are usually the lower risk types, less likely to lead to precancers and cancers. If you have developed genital warts and are in a monogamous relationship, discuss this with your partner. You should obtain a detailed sexual history from him or her. You may want to consider being tested for other sexually transmitted diseases and discuss treatment options with your health care provider.

37. Can I give genital warts to my partner?

Yes, it is possible. Unfortunately, because most people are unaware that they have HPV, they are not actively working to prevent transmission. Transmission of HPV is best prevented by refraining from sexual contact, which is 100% effective in preventing sexually transmitted diseases in general. Because that is not a viable option for most people, using latex condoms is the next best answer. Condoms are not 100% effective, as the virus may be present in uncovered areas.

Genital warts are contagious, as they shed HPV. Almost all genital warts are transmitted through sexual contact, and thus, you need to be most concerned with your intimate partner. Genital warts in men are often not visible to the naked eye and may be tiny or within the urethra or under the foreskin in an uncircumcised partner. Condoms provide some degree of protection; however, as there is still skin-to-skin contact during sexual contact, they are not 100% protective. Theoretically, genital warts may rarely be transmitted by more casual nonsexual contact, although this isn't known with certainty. Practicing good hygiene, including hand washing after any hand contact with one's own genital area, or after using the bathroom, is an appropriate measure.

Almost all genital warts are transmitted through sexual contact, and thus, you need to be most concerned with your intimate partner.

HPV can be transmitted even if you don't see any warts. Warts may not be visible without magnification. Also, HPV can be present in normal-appearing skin, and the virus can shed. Visible genital warts are more common in women than men, however, and the cervix is more vulnerable to premalignant and malignant conditions associated with HPV than the penis or anus in men; therefore, it is important for women to protect themselves. The use of condoms offers some, but not total, protection. The types of HPV that cause warts are considered to be "low-risk," with a low chance of causing cervical or vulvar cancers or precancers. The high-risk types of HPV associated with these cancers and precancers don't usually cause visible warts.

38. Can I give it to my partner if I don't have warts?

Yes. Even if you are infected but don't have warts, you can still give HPV to your sexual partner. Genital warts can be acquired during oral, vaginal, or anal sex with any infected partner. You can also get them by skin-to-skin contact during vaginal, anal, or oral sex with someone who is infected. About two thirds of people who have sexual contact with a partner with genital warts will develop warts themselves. The warts usually appear within 3 months of the initial contact, but time can be very variable.

39. I have heard a lot about the HPV vaccine. What is a vaccine?

A **vaccine** is a substance that stimulates the body's immune response, causing the body to produce disease-preventing or disease-fighting antibodies. The goal of vaccination is to prevent or control an infection. Usually, a specific vaccine is designed to prevent a specific disease. There are different types of vaccines. The type of vaccine used depends on which disease it is targeted to prevent or control. A vaccine may be aimed at preventing a disease (a **prophylactic** vaccine) or fighting a disease that you already have (a therapeutic vaccine). Most vaccines you have received in your life are prophylactic.

Vaccine

A substance that stimulates the body's immune response, causing the body to produce disease-preventing or disease-fighting antibodies. The goal of vaccination is to prevent or control an infection. Usually, a specific vaccine is designed to prevent a specific disease.

Prophylactic

Preventive or protective.

Human papilloma virus vaccine

Recently developed to prevent the transmission of certain types of the human papilloma virus, thereby reducing the chances of getting cervical cancer.

40. What is the HPV vaccine?

The **HPV vaccine** prevents the transmission of certain types of HPV. It was designed to target the most common high-risk types, which are known to cause cervical cancer; however, at least one HPV vaccine also targets the low-risk types of HPV that cause genital warts. Studies have found the vaccine to be almost 100% effective in preventing diseases caused by the HPV types covered by the vaccine, including precancers of the cervix, vulva, and vagina and genital warts in women with a low risk of having already contracted the virus. The vaccine is not meant to treat patients who already have HPV-related conditions. The vaccine has mainly been studied in young women who have not been exposed to any of the HPV types in the vaccine. This vaccine does not treat existing HPV infections, genital warts, precancers, or cancers.

Studies have found the vaccine to be almost 100% effective in preventing diseases caused by the HPV types covered by the vaccine, including precancers of the cervix, vulva, and vagina and genital warts in women with a low risk of having already contracted the virus.

Recombinant

A recombinant vaccine contains a substance that stimulates the immune system without containing viral DNA.

Approximately 30% of cervical cancers will *not* be prevented by the vaccine, as they are caused by other HPV types; thus, it is important that women continue to get screened for cervical cancer with regular Pap smears. Also, the vaccine does *not* prevent about 10% of genital warts—nor will it prevent other sexually transmitted diseases.

The vaccine is **recombinant**, which means that it will not give you HPV, as it does not contain any infectious material. HPV vaccines are essentially a suit of clothes with no body inside that fools the body into making a defense against this "invader."

Ellen comments:

Even though it may seem premature to think about it, I discussed the HPV vaccine for my young daughter with my gynecologist at my last annual visit. She said that I did have time to think about this but that it was good that I was thinking ahead, especially because, ideally, girls would get the vaccine before they become sexually active. There are so few side effects of the vaccine, and they are rare. At her (my daughter's) next visit with the pediatrician, I am going to tell him to plan for her to be vaccinated when the time comes.

41. Am I eligible for it?

The HPV vaccine is recommended for 11- to 12-year-old girls and can be given to girls as young as 9-years-old. The vaccine is also recommended for 13- to 26-year-old women who have not yet received or completed the vaccine series. It is not recommended for pregnant women. The ideal vaccination period is for the younger girl who is not yet sexually active and hence has not been sexually exposed to HPV.

We do not yet know whether the vaccine is effective in boys or men. Vaccinating males might have health benefits by preventing genital warts and rare cancers, such as penile and anal cancer. It is also possible that vaccinating men will have indirect health benefits for women, thus decreasing spread. Studies are now being done to find out whether the vaccine works to prevent HPV infection and disease in males. Studies in women over 26 years old are also underway to see whether there is any benefit in women who have more than likely already been exposed to HPV.

Alanna comments:

The answer depends on you and your child. The reality is that many girls are becoming sexually active at a younger age. Some parents may not feel comfortable discussing sexuality with their 9-year-old and feel that they are too young to have these discussions. Other parents may view getting the vaccine as an opportunity to discuss safe sex practices with their daughters. Ultimately, you know your child better than anyone else, and it is a decision that should be tailored to each child.

42. How are genital warts treated?

Genital warts can be treated with a medication that the patient applies at home or by treatments applied by a health care provider in the office. The method that is used depends on patient preference, the experience of the health care provider, the size, shape, and number of the warts, their anatomic location, and treatment cost. No single treatment is superior to another but rather depends on the patients and the wart(s). In fact, given that some warts will resolve on their own, some women prefer not to receive treatment and wait to see whether the warts resolve. Most warts require a few treatment sessions, rather than a single treatment. Most genital warts respond within 3 months of therapy.

Most warts require a few treatment sessions, rather than a single treatment. Most genital warts respond within 3 months of therapy.

There are a variety of ways in which genital warts can be treated. None of them are completely effective, and recurrences are common. Depending on the location of the warts, the number of warts, and provider and patient preference, some medications may be applied in the privacy of the home, whereas some require visits to a provider. Therapy is aimed at eradicating the warts and modifying the regional immune response. Patient-applied therapies include **imiquimod** and **podofilox** 0.5%, the active component of **podophyllin**. Larger warts may be removed surgically, but other treatments are designed to destroy (ablate) the warts but do not provide an excised specimen for histologic evaluation (by the **pathologist**). Ablative therapies include application of podophyllin, which is performed in the doctor's office, although there is a weaker formulation that can be used at home, podofilox. Care must be taken, as podophyllin and podofilox can cause birth defects, and pregnancy must be prevented during their use. Another ablative treatment, **trichloroacetic acid**, also requires office visits. Both trichloroacetic acid and podophyllin can be very irritating to normal skin, although contact with the normal skin is something the provider will try to prevent. **Cryotherapy** (freezing) and laser therapy are other options. Laser ablation therapy of the wart may be done as an outpatient surgical procedure or in the clinician's office. Although complications are uncommon, skin changes, such as decreased or increased pigmentation, are common with laser therapy.

Imiquimod

Used to treat external genital and anal warts (*condyloma accuminata*).

Podofilox

A medication used to treat genital warts.

Podophyllin

A topical medication used to treat external genital warts.

Pathologist

A doctor who studies the origin, nature, and course of diseases.

Trichloroacetic acid

Used in a diluted form to treat genital warts.

Cryotherapy

A method of treating external genital warts by freezing them.

More recently, the immune modifier imiquimod has had some success in this area, and patients may apply it at home. It is not approved for use during pregnancy. Injection of interferon into the warts has also been used as an immune modifier. All of the available treatments are associated with some degree of discomfort. Also, HPV, like HSV, remains in the body even after therapy; thus, recurrences requiring retreatment are not rare. Treatments applied in the provider's office, such as trichloroacetic acid, usually require a few sessions. Prescription topical creams and gels such as imiquimod or podofilox that are applied a few times a week by the patient at home for several weeks are often a favored form of therapy. For treatment to be effective, the patient must be compliant in using the medication appropriately, however, and must be able to identify and reach all genital warts. Rarely, chronic pain syndromes may occur at the treatment site with any of these treatments.

When left untreated, visible genital warts may resolve spontaneously, remain unchanged, or increase in size or number. The goal of treating genital warts is to remove them, which in most patients can induce wart-free periods. Treatment possibly reduces but does not eliminate HPV infection, and it is not clear whether treatment impacts future transmission. It is important to understand that the presence of genital warts and/or their treatment is almost never associated with the development of cervical cancer.

Many different types of HPV can affect the vulva. The ones that cause genital warts, most often HPV types 6 and 11, are considered low-risk types, not likely to progress to a cancer. Most HPV-associated vulvar cancers are associated with one of the high-risk types of HPV, such as HPV 16, 18, and 31.

Mary's comments:

I was diagnosed with warts several years ago. I didn't know I had them until I got pregnant and registered for prenatal care. When my doctor told me I had two warts, I was horrified. She explained that they could be easily taken care of and that they would not affect the baby. I went to her every week, and she put a little bit of acid on the warts each time. After a few weeks, they were gone. I went on to delivery a healthy baby girl, and I have not had another wart since then.

43. What is HPV?

HPV stands for human papilloma virus. It is a DNA virus that affects skin and mucous membranes. Over 100 types are known, not all of which affect the genital tract. Some cause the common skin wart, medically known as **verruca vulgaris**. Plantar warts, on the soles of the feet, are from a different type of HPV. Some HPV types affect the external genital tract of both men and women. Some of these, the low-risk types, such as HPV 6 and 11, are associated with genital warts (condyloma acuminatum) and rarely are a cancer risk. HPV may affect the external genitalia (the vulva, perineum, and perianal skin), as well as the internal genitalia such as the cervix, vagina, urethra, and anus. HPV types 6 and 11 have also been associated with conjunctival, nasal, oral, and laryngeal warts, although these are less common.

Verruca vulgaris
The common skin wart.

HPV may affect the external genitalia (the vulva, perineum, and perianal skin), as well as the internal genitalia such as the cervix, vagina, urethra, and anus.

Some of the genital types of HPV infect the skin and mucosa of the vulvar region but produce no noticeable disease. Some of the HPV types can cause precancerous lesions that eventually progress to cancerous lesions of the lower genital tract. These HPV types are divided into intermediate- and high-risk types. Lesions may affect the vulva, vagina, and cervix in women, the penis in men, and the perianal area in both sexes. Infection with HPV is extremely common in sexually active adults, and more than half of all women are likely to contract the virus at some point in their lives. Hence, it is important to get routine Pap smears to detect the early cervical cellular abnormalities that can be associated with HPV; then appropriate follow-up and any necessary treatment can be instituted. Most cases of HPV related cancers can be prevented. Adjunct testing for the virus is sometimes performed at the same time as a Pap smear in women over 30 years old to guide management. More than half the women who contract HPV will spontaneously clear the virus from their systems within 2 years. Because of the high prevalence of HPV in women under 30 years of age and the high clearance rate, routine testing for the virus is not recommended for those less than 30 years old. It is the persistence of the virus, not merely infection with the virus, that is the risk factor for precancers and cancers. By not routinely testing younger women for the virus, it is hoped to avoid overly vigorous interventions in this age group; however, it is one of the acceptable screening modalities in women over the age of 30. Nevertheless, young women still need Pap smears!

HPV is transmitted sexually by skin-to-skin contact as well as mucosal contact; hence, although condoms will offer some protection, they are not entirely effective in preventing transmission. More than half of all sexually active women encounter HPV; however, few get cervical cancer, and vulvar cancer is even rarer.

44. Can I give it to my children?

There are three ways that HPV can be transmitted: sexual transmission, vertical transmission, and horizontal transmission. Sexual transmission is by far the most common method of spreading HPV. Hence, when a child develops genital warts, the possibility of abuse is raised; however, this is not felt to be true in all cases, although it should trigger an investigation. In vertical transmission, the virus is transmitted to the infant when it passes through the birth canal (vagina). Although many infants are exposed to HPV in this manner, actual disease manifestations are extremely rare. One serious sequela, **laryngeal papillomatosis**, is the development of warty growths in the respiratory tract of the child, including the larynx. Rarely, it can spread to the lungs. Laryngeal papillomas can block the flow of air in the trachea (wind pipe), causing severe respiratory problems, and the disease is characteristically one of repeated recurrences after treatment. Laser therapy is used in treating this condition. Luckily, it is exceptionally rare, and most children born of mothers with HPV have no related problems. You likely have never heard of anyone with laryngeal papillomatosis, yet if up to 75% of sexually active women have been exposed to HPV, you definitely know people who have been exposed! Horizontal transmission of HPV refers to the spread of HPV via nonsexual contact such as from the hands of infected caregivers that come in contact with the external genitalia of an infant during diapering or from adult to adult via **fomites** (such as towels). HPV has been found on the fingertips of adults with genital HPV, and thus, it may be spread to a child via an activity like diaper changing, although this has not been conclusively proven. Hand washing after use of the bathroom is always a good idea. HPV has not been shown to be transmissible by a toilet seat.

Laryngeal papillomatosis

A condition characterized by multiple squamous cell papillomas of the larynx, seen most commonly in young children, usually due to infection by the human papilloma virus transmitted at birth from maternal genital warts.

Fomites

Any agent, such as clothing or bedding, that is capable of absorbing and transmitting the infecting organism of a disease.

Genital warts may become problematic during pregnancy because they can multiply and grow. Depending on the size and location, they may need to be removed before delivery to ensure a safe and healthy delivery of the newborn. If the warts get large enough, it may be difficult to urinate if the warts obstruct the urethra, the tube that drains the bladder and opens into the vestibule. If the warts are in the vagina, they can cause obstruction during delivery and bleed during childbirth.

45. *Will it affect my fertility?*

HPV or genital warts will not directly affect fertility; however, some of the therapies associated with treatment of preinvasive cervical lesions may cause some difficulty. Procedures that involve resecting significant amounts of cervical tissue, such as a **cone biopsy**, may lead to scarring of the cervix. This can cause difficulty with cervical dilation at the time of delivery and may result in a higher chance of a cesarean delivery. Alternatively, the cervix may not be able to remain closed throughout a pregnancy after some procedures, resulting in an incompetent cervix, a condition of painless dilation and premature pregnancy loss. Thus, routine screening for HPV is not recommended in women under 30 years who are likely to be interested in fertility. This is to avoid causing these potential complications of pregnancy among women by overzealous treatment of low-grade lesions that have a good chance of regressing by themselves. High-grade lesions still need to be treated, and low-grade lesions still need to be followed; therefore, if you get one of these diagnoses, ask questions, but be sure to follow up with your healthcare provider. Becoming pregnant is not affected by HPV; however, as is the case in any sexually transmitted disease, it is always possible to have more than one, simply by the increased risk of exposure, and chlamydia or gonorrhea can lead to difficulties conceiving because of scarring of the fallopian tubes.

Cone biopsy

Refers to a surgical procedure to remove part of the female cervix.

There are three ways that HPV can be transmitted: sexual transmission, vertical transmission, and horizontal transmission.

46. *Do genital warts cause vulvar cancer?*

Many different types of HPV can affect the vulva. The ones that cause genital warts, most often HPV types 6 and 11, are considered low-risk types, not likely to progress to a cancer. Most HPV-associated vulvar cancers are associated with one of the high-risk types of HPV, such as HPV 16, 18, and 31. The high-risk types do not commonly cause warts. Strains of the HPV that have been linked to cervical and vulvar cancer are different from the ones that usually cause external genital warts. HPV types 16, 18, 31, 33, and 35 are associated with "squamous **intraepithelial neoplasia**" (a precancer) of the external genitalia, vagina, or cervix, as opposed to HPV types 6 and 11, which are linked to external warts. Sometimes (but not always), a precancer may progress to a cervical or vulvar cancer. Thus, getting regular Pap smears and examinations is very important. It usually takes a few years for precancer to develop into cancer. Most cervical and vulvar precancers that are caused by HPV are easily treated, and thus, with Pap smears and examinations, cervical and vulvar cancers are largely preventable diseases!

Intraepithelial neoplasia

Also known as cervical dysplasia, a potentially premalignant transformation and abnormal growth (dysplasia) of squamous cells on the surface of the cervix.

47. What other sexually transmitted diseases can occur on the vulva?

A variety of conditions can occur on the vulva; these may present as lumps or bumps. **Tables 3–13** list some of these conditions, but are not all inclusive. These conditions can be put into broad categories, including sexually transmitted diseases, nonsexually transmitted inflammatory or infectious conditions (not all conditions associated with inflammation are contagious, also termed infectious), many of which are dermatologic in nature, nonneoplastic epithelial disorders, benign **neoplasms** (tumors), and malignant neoplasms (tumors).

Neoplasm

A new, often uncontrolled growth of abnormal tissue.

Sexually Transmitted Diseases

Syphilis, HIV, gonorrhea, chlamydia, and herpes, in addition to HPV, are the most commonly encountered sexually transmitted diseases in developed nations. Granuloma inguinale, lymphogranuloma venereum, and chancroid, all of which may present as a swelling or an ulcer at some point in their evolution, are uncommon in the United States. Gonorrhea and chlamydia may be silent (asymptomatic) in women and not become apparent until there is scarring of the fallopian tubes, with resultant infertility. Sometimes they present with vaginal discharge or if the infection has spread to pelvic organs **pelvic inflammatory disease**. Sexually active individuals should practice safer sex at every sexual encounter and should be honest in disclosing their sexual practices to their practitioners so that appropriate counseling, screening, and treatment can be performed. Although the only guaranteed form of prevention of sexually transmitted diseases is abstinence, the use of condoms has greatly reduced, but not eliminated, their spread. Although the following is not meant to be an exhaustive discussion of sexually transmitted diseases, aspects relating to presentation on the vulva are discussed. Further information on a variety of sexually transmitted diseases is available on the Centers for Disease Control website at *http://www.cdc.gov/std/healthcomm/fact_sheets.htm*. It has been shown that the presence of some of the discussed sexually transmitted diseases increases the risk of acquiring HIV after a sexual exposure to an HIV-positive partner.

Pelvic inflammatory disease

A term used to describe any infection in the lower female reproductive tract that spreads to the upper female reproductive tract.

Syphilis

A resurgence of syphilis has occurred in our population. Syphilis is caused by an organism called treponema pallidum. The initial presenting lesion is a **chancre**, which is a painless ulcer with raised edges, occurring on the genitalia, anus, or mouth. If untreated, primary syphilis

Chancre

The initial lesion of syphilis, commonly a more or less distinct ulcer or sore with distinct edges.

can progress to secondary or tertiary syphilis. Secondary syphilis shows up as a rash and lesions of the mucous membranes. Tertiary syphilis can affect and damage a variety of organs. Syphilis may be silent for many years and later present with internal damage to a variety of organs, including the heart and brain. The best way to prevent syphilis is to either abstain from sex or be in a relationship in which both partners are free of sexually transmitted diseases and are monogamous. Condom use cuts down on the risk of transmission but does not eliminate it entirely. Syphilis is treated with antibiotics. Partners must be tested and treated if needed. Syphilis can affect a fetus with varying degrees of damage.

Table 3 Sexually Transmitted Diseases Affecting the Vulva

Syphilis
Gonorrhea
Chlamydia
Herpes
Granuloma inguinale
Lymphogranuloma venereum
Chancroid
HPV
HIV

Table 4 Inflammatory Dermatoses Affecting the Vulva

Eczema
Psoriasis
Lichen planus
Zoon's vulvitis
Crohn's disease
Hidradenitis suppurativa
Aphthae
- *Benign*
- *Behçet's syndrome*

Autoimmune bullous dermatoses
- *Pemphigoid, Linear IgA, Pemphigus*

Table 5 Infectious Diseases Affecting the Vulva

Varicella zoster
Molluscum contagiosum
Tuberculosis
Staphylococcus aureus
Candidiasis
Tinea cruris
Scabies
Pubic lice

Table 6 Nonneoplastic Epithelial Disorders (ISSVD, 1987)

Lichen sclerosus
Squamous cell hyperplasia
Other dermatoses

Table 7 Cysts of the Vulva

Bartholin's gland cyst and abscess
Epidermal inclusion cyst
Less common benign cysts:
- Mucinous and ciliated cysts
- Mesonephric-like cyst (Wolffian duct-like cyst)
- Cyst of the canal of Nuck (mesothelial cyst)

Table 8 Some Benign Tumor-Like Lesions of the Vulva

Vestibular adenosis
Endometriosis
Fibroepithelial polyp (acrochordon, or skin tag)
Micropapillomatosis labialis

Table 9 Some Benign Neoplasms Affecting the Vulva

Lesions of the glands around the hair follicles
- Papillary hidradenoma (hidradenoma papilliferum)
- Trichoepithelioma
- Syringoma

Lesions of the squamous epithelium lining the vulva
- Seborrheic keratosis
- Warty dyskeratoma
- Keratoacanthoma
- Angiokeratoma
- Pyogenic granuloma (granuloma pyogenicum)

(*continues*)

Table 9 Some Benign Neoplasms Affecting the Vulva (Continued)

Lesions of the connective tissue under the skin
Dermatofibroma
Hemangioma
Lymphangioma circumscriptum
Angiomyofibroblastoma
Aggressive angiomyxoma
Granular cell tumor
Leiomyoma
Fibroma
Lipoma
Mammary tissue within vulva
Neurofibroma

Table 10 Preinvasive (In Situ) Neoplasms of the Vulva

Vulvar intraepithelial neoplasia (VIN)
Differentiated VIN
Paget's disease of the vulva
Melanoma in situ

Table 11 More Common Invasive Neoplasms of the Vulva

Squamous cell carcinoma
Verrucous carcinoma
Melanoma
Basal cell carcinoma
Bartholin's gland carcinoma
Invasive Paget's disease

Table 12 Lesions of the Urethra and Adjacent Structures*

Urethral prolapse
Urethral caruncle
Malacoplakia of the urethra
Paraurethral (Skene's duct) cyst
Suburethral diverticulum
Leiomyoma of the urethra
Urethral carcinoma

* Benign except for carcinoma

Table 13 Pigmented Lesions of the Vulva

- Acanthosis nigricans
- Melanocytic lesions
  - Melanosis
  - Benign nevi (moles)
  - Atypical junctional melanocytic hyperplasia
  - Melanoma in situ
  - Melanoma

Gonorrhea

Gonorrhea, caused by *Neisseria gonorrhoeae*, is very common. Although men often present with burning on urination and a penile yellowish discharge, women often have few or no symptoms. When present, symptoms include vaginal discharge, irregular bleeding, or burning on urination. Regardless of whether gonorrhea is initially symptomatic, it can go on to pelvic inflammatory disease, infertility, and risk of tubal ectopic pregnancy in women. Pelvic inflammatory disease is inflammation of the fallopian tubes, possibly ovaries, and lining tissue of the pelvis and presents with fever and pelvic pain, although it may be silent. Gonorrhea is treated with antibiotics. Partners must be evaluated and treated as necessary. As with other sexually transmitted diseases, condoms can decrease transmission markedly.

Chlamydia

Chlamydia is more common than gonorrhea. It is caused by an organism called chlamydia trachomatis. It presents with symptoms that are similar to gonorrhea or a lack of symptoms in women, and it can also result in silent damage to the fallopian tubes with resultant infertility and a risk of tubal ectopic pregnancy. In an era when women often delay having their families to pursue a career, it is unfortunate that some of them discover very

The risk of contracting a sexually transmitted disease is related to the risk of one's partners and all of their partners.

late that they have residual damage to fallopian tubes and are unable to conceive spontaneously. Chlamydia is treated with antibiotics. Partners must be evaluated and treated as necessary. As with other sexually transmitted diseases, condoms can decrease transmission markedly.

Herpes

For a more detailed discussion on herpes, see Questions 25–29.

Herpes on the vulva is usually caused by HSV-2 but can be caused by HSV-1 as well. It is usually sexually transmitted but can also be spread by oral–genital contact. Herpes is a very common genital infection, and most people who have it do not know that they do. The initial outbreak can be very symptomatic, with multiple blisters that rupture and become painful sores and flu-like symptoms. Urination may be particularly painful when urine touches the sores; however, recurrent episodes are markedly less severe and decrease in frequency over time. People with genital herpes may not be aware of an outbreak, and the virus may be shed from normal appearing skin. Hence, herpes may be contagious even in the absence of an outbreak or visible lesions. Condoms provide some protection, but herpes can be transmitted through uncovered skin. Although people who have genital herpes often suffer psychologic stress associated with the condition, it is extremely common in the population and should not be taken as a sign of having done something "bad" or inappropriate. The most severe potential consequence is transmitting herpes to a newborn during delivery, as a herpes infection may be fatal to the infant. Newly acquired active herpes at the time of the delivery may be particularly severe. Cesarean deliveries are often performed if the mother has an active genital herpes sore at the time of delivery, depending on the clinical circumstances. Herpes cannot be cured, but suppressive therapy is available.

Herpes is a very common genital infection, and most people who have it do not know that they do. The initial outbreak can be very symptomatic, with multiple blisters that rupture and become painful sores and flu-like symptoms.

Granuloma Inguinale, Lymphogranuloma Venereum, and Chancroid

Granuloma inguinale, lymphogranuloma venereum, and chancroid are more common in tropical locales, although they do occur in the United States. These conditions may present with a variety of ulcerations and/or groin swellings. Chancroid in particular is known for having painful ulcers, whereas most of the other ulcerating sexually transmitted diseases are painless.

Tests are available that can tell you whether you have a specific sexually transmitted disease, and effective treatments are available for all sexually transmitted diseases, although HIV is not curable. If you have a sexually transmitted disease, seek immediate treatment. Although you have been treated, you can still get the sexually transmitted disease again; therefore, your partner should be tested and treated (if needed) as well.

Benign or malignant (cancerous) growths can look like a genital wart. Benign growths include skin tags, inclusion cysts, and other dermatologic conditions such as a mole. Premalignant conditions include vulvar or vaginal intraepithelial neoplasia (see Question 61), which may progress onto a vulvar or vaginal cancer if not treated.

48. How do I protect myself from sexually transmitted diseases?

The number of people affected by sexually transmitted diseases has been increasing in the past 20 years. This occurs because young people are becoming sexually active at earlier ages and marrying later. Additionally, sexually active people typically have more than one sexual partner during their lifetime. The risk of contracting a sexually transmitted disease is related to the risk of one's partners and all of their partners.

Frequently, sexually transmitted diseases do not cause symptoms, especially in women. To make matters worse, when and if symptoms develop, they may be confused with symptoms of other diseases that are not actually sexually transmitted diseases. Thus, even if you don't have symptoms of a sexually transmitted disease, you can still transmit it to another person; therefore, the best way to protect yourself is to not engage in sexual activity unless you are certain your partner does not have a sexually transmitted disease. If you are not sure, a latex condom provides the best protection, although it is not 100% effective. Natural (lambskin) condoms are effective at preventing pregnancy but are not be as effective in preventing the transmission of sexually transmitted diseases.

Because sexually active women can be especially asymptomatic and not know that they have an infection and thus can pass it onto other people, getting tested is very important. Talk with your health care provider about getting tested for sexually transmitted diseases, particularly if you have more than one sexual partner. Be honest with your provider—they are there to help, not judge, you. You don't have to have symptoms to get tested!

49. What other lumps and bumps can occur on the vulva?

Inflammatory Dermatoses

A variety of noninfectious, noncontagious inflammatory conditions can occur on the vulva, which is a dermatologic as well as a gynecologic organ. A dermatologist with a special interest in the vulva is able to treat these conditions,and some gynecologists are also particularly focused on vulvar diseases. In addition, some dermatologic conditions, such as **eczema**, **psoriasis**, or the bullous or blistering dermatoses, that can affect the skin anywhere can also affect the vulva. There are conditions unique to the region, such as Zoon's vulvitis (also called plasma cell vulvitis); this condition is quite rare and thus is not discussed further. Diseases affecting other areas of the body can have specific vulvar manifestations, such as **Crohn's disease** or lichen planus. **Hidradenitis suppurativa** also affects the axillary region (the armpit) and can be quite severe on the vulva, often requiring surgical intervention. Gynecologists and dermatologists with special interest or expertise in the vulva usually see the vulvar hidradenitis patients. A gynecologist would be the one to perform any surgery needed.

Eczema

An inflammatory condition of the skin attended with itching and the exudation of serous matter.

Psoriasis

A common chronic inflammatory skin disease characterized by scaly patches.

Crohn's disease

A chronic inflammatory disease of the bowel that may cause scarring and thickening of the intestinal walls and frequently leads to obstruction.

Hidradenitis suppurativa

An inflammatory condition that affects regions of the body containing sweat glands such as the armpit, under the breasts, in the creases of the thighs, buttocks, and vulva. It is more common in women, particularly those who are obese. Draining pustules, abscesses, blackheads, and swellings ("boils") characterize the condition, which can cause a great deal of distress.

A number of these conditions may present as itching. Not all itching is caused by a yeast infection, as women often assume. If itching is persistent, evaluation by a health care provider should be sought, as many treatments are available. Itching may be caused by one of a variety of dermatologic conditions such as an infection, or it may be due to contact dermatitis, which is an irritation from a product used, or an actual allergy to a product. Reactions to products, irritant or allergic, may range from mild itching to redness to blisters and weeping, with crusts and even bleeding. Appropriate vulvar hygiene and care are important. This includes avoiding potentially irritating products in the area; wearing loose clothing, cotton underwear, and cotton pads or tampons; and avoiding overwashing/scrubbing in the area. Some people may be allergic to latex condoms and are sensitive or allergic to a variety of feminine hygiene products. Further information on contact dermatitis can be found at *http://www.nlm.nih.gov/medlineplus/ency/article/000869.htm*.

Eczema

Eczema can affect the skin anywhere on the body, including the vulva. It may be red or scaly, and it is very itchy. With scratching, the vulvar skin may develop swelling and cracks and may become thickened. The most common form of eczema, called atopic eczema, is an allergic condition. It may be associated with other allergies and may have some familial tendency. A provider can recommend a variety of topical therapies, including steroidal preparations for the treatment of eczema. Further information can be found at *http://www.nlm.nih.gov/medlineplus/eczema.html.*

Psoriasis

Psoriasis, often found on the elbows, can also affect the vulva. It is a common condition, and the cause is not known. It may burn or itch. The redness is well demarcated, and it may be scaly in appearance, with silvery scales on top of red areas, although in the vulvar region psoriasis tends to be red and moist. The scales associated with psoriasis are caused by skin that is regenerating too quickly, and thus, it sheds in scales. It is not contagious. It can't be cured, but can be effectively managed and controlled. In addition to the previously discussed general vulvar hygiene, a variety of topical therapies may be prescribed. See *http://www.nlm.nih.gov/medlineplus/psoriasis.html* for further information.

Lichen Planus

Lichen planus is discussed in detail in Question 58. It may affect the vulva, and it might be diagnosed from involvement of the mouth and eye. Your provider should examine inside your mouth and in your eye area if this is suspected. Lichen planus may cause the skin to be red, with white streaks. It may be erosive, thus causing pain and making intercourse difficult because of scarring inside the vagina. A variety of therapies, including topical steroids, retinoids, tacrolimus, and methotrexate, have been used. The histology is distinct, and a biopsy may be needed to make the diagnosis. For further information, see *http://www.nlm.nih.gov/medlineplus/ency/article/000867.htm*.

Crohn's Disease

Crohn's disease is a type of inflammatory bowel disease that can occasionally present on the vulva of affected individuals. When it does, it may be direct extension of the inflammation from the bowel or may be a secondary separate site of inflammation. The vulva may simply be swollen, but ulcers, abscesses, and fistulas (tissue tracts) may be present. A biopsy may be needed to make the diagnosis. See *http://www.nlm.nih.gov/medlineplus/crohnsdisease.html* for further information.

Hidradenitis Suppurativa

Hidradenitis suppurativa is an inflammatory condition that affects regions of the body containing apocrine sweat glands, and hence, the armpit, under the breasts, and in the creases of the thighs, buttocks, and vulva are favored sites in women. It is more common in women, particularly in those who are obese. Draining pustules, abscesses, blackheads, and swellings ("boils") characterize the condition. These can cause a great deal of distress. Although medication may manage less severe cases, the more severe ones may come to surgical excision, sometimes with a skin graft.

Rare Inflammatory Conditions

Other rare conditions include **aphthae**, ulcers that may be isolated or present in the mouth, usually in children, or may be part of Behçet's syndrome, a rare multisystem disorder that involves the mouth and eyes and can involve

Aphthae

Another word for a canker sore.

other organs and is recurrent. Autoimmune bullous dermatoses present as blisters, and specialized testing of the blisters, which requires a biopsy, may be needed to render a diagnosis. Further information can be found on Behçet's syndrome at *http://www.nlm.nih.gov/medlineplus/behcetssyndrome.html* and on the bullous dermatoses at *http://www.aad.org/public/publications/pamphlets/common_bullous.html.*

Molluscum contagiosum

A virus disease of the skin marked by round white swellings; transmitted from person to person (most often in children or in adults with impaired immune function).

Tinea cruris

A fungal infection of the skin of the groin area, occurring more commonly in warm weather and characterized by red ring-like areas, sometimes with small blisters, and severe itching.

Scabies

A contagious skin disease caused by the itch mite, *Sarcoptes scabiei*, which burrows under the skin.

Pubic lice

Small, six-legged parasites that infect the genital hair area and lay eggs.

Infectious Diseases

A variety of nonsexually transmitted infectious (sometimes contagious) diseases can affect the vulva. They are caused by different bacteria (tuberculosis, *Staphylococcus aureus*), viruses (varicella zoster, [chickenpox or shingles], **molluscum contagiosum**), fungi (*candidiasis*, **tinea cruris**), and parasites (**scabies**, **pubic lice**). A brief discussion of the more common infections follows.

Molluscum Contagiosum

In the adult, molluscum presents on the genital region, abdomen, and thighs and is usually sexually transmitted; however, molluscum contagiosum is common in children and can involve the entire body. In these cases, it is spread by skin-to-skin contact and is not considered to be a sexually transmitted disease in children in the majority of cases. The lesions are small raised bumps with a central umbilication or indentation that can be expressed. There are often no symptoms, or the lesions can be itchy. The lesions often resolve on their own in up to 2 years, but your health care provider can use a variety of treatments. Destruction of the lesions, expression of the contents by scraping, and treatment with topical imiquimod have been used. The lesions may be larger and more difficult to treat in immunosuppressed patients.

Staphylococcus Aureus

The range of staphylococcal infections affecting the vulva is from the minor infected hair follicles seen after shaving (folliculitis), to boils, to severe infections requiring hospitalization, to toxic shock syndrome if the bacteria produce the syndrome-causing toxins. Treatment of minor infections can be local, including topical compresses, drainage, in addition to antibiotics, but severe infections require hospitalization.

Candidiasis

Although candida ("yeast infection") is best known for producing the characteristic itchy white "cottage-cheese" vaginal discharge, the vulvar skin may be affected as well, in which case it is red and itchy and may be sore. This is more common in diabetic and obese women, as well as in the face of fecal or urinary incontinence or **immunosuppression**. Although many women think that all infections and discharges are yeast infections, this should be confirmed by culture or microscopy, particularly if recurrent. A variety of topical or oral medications are available to treat vulvar candidiasis.

Immunosuppression

The inhibition of the normal immune response because of disease, the administration of drugs, or surgery.

Tinea Cruris

Tinea cruris is better known as "jock itch." It is more common in men who are obese and in individuals who also have athlete's foot. It can occur on the inner thighs and the creases of the groins and on the vulva, and it is marked by an itchy rash. It is usually treated by topical medications but may require oral medications if the fungus has tracked down into the hair follicles. Diagnosis is by examining scrapings under the microscope or by culture or by response to therapy.

Scabies

Scabies is caused by a microscopic-sized mite and is contracted through skin-to-skin contact. It can be transmitted sexually or nonsexually and has nothing to do with uncleanliness. The mite burrows under the skin, causing severe itching, particularly at night. It is usually treated topically. Household members are also usually treated, and linens and clothing must be washed in hot, soapy water and dried in a hot dryer, dry cleaned, or bagged for 2 weeks to eliminate the mites. For further information, see *http://www.aad.org/public/publications/pamphlets/common_scabies.html.*

Pubic Lice

Pubic lice are known as the "crabs" and can be transmitted sexually or by fomites (bedding, towels, etc.). They are annoying and cause itching. Treatment is usually topical. The fomites must be treated by washing or bagging for 2 weeks and eliminating the nits (eggs) with a special comb. See *http://www.nlm.nih.gov/medlineplus/ency/article/000841.htm.*

Nonneoplastic Epithelial Disorders

This term was coined by the International Society for the Study of Vulvovaginal Diseases in 1987 to cover a variety of conditions recognized by specific histologic features that had previously been called the vulvar dystrophies. It was recognized that these conditions were not dystrophic (degenerative) and hence the replaced terminology, which now consists of lichen sclerosus, **squamous cell hyperplasia**, and other dermatoses.

Squamous cell hyperplasia

An irregular white or gray patch of the skin of the vulva that is slightly raised (thickened).

Lichen Sclerosus

Lichen sclerosus used to be called "lichen sclerosus et atrophicus" because of the thin appearance of the vulvar skin, which becomes thin or "atrophic," white, and wrinkly, associated with severe itching. This thin white appearance has been termed "cigarette paper," but in spite of the appearance, the condition is not one of atrophy. There is some hereditary component to the disease, which can be seen over the bodies as well as in a vulvar location in children, but is usually seen on the vulva in older white women. It is unclear whether having lichen sclerosus is a risk factor for developing vulvar **carcinoma** (squamous cell carcinoma). There have been reports of squamous cell carcinoma of the vulva occurring in association with vulvar lichen sclerosus, but it is still not known whether the two are related or coincidental. Vulvar squamous cell carcinoma is not a common condition, and thus, collecting large enough numbers of cases to get some useful information on risk is difficult. In any case, because it is unclear what the risk is and because of the potential complications of lichen sclerosus, it is important to receive ongoing care from a health care provider for this chronic condition. If untreated, lichen sclerosus can lead to scarring of the vulva, with narrowing of the vaginal opening, which can interfere with sexual activity. There can be alteration of the anatomy, with loss of the labia minora and burying of the clitoris. Topical treatment with ultra potent prescription topical steroids can manage the condition, but not cure it.

Carcinoma

An invasive malignant tumor derived from epithelial tissue that tends to metastasize to other areas of the body.

Squamous Cell Hyperplasia

Squamous cell hyperplasia (also called lichen simplex chronicus) is a thickening of the vulvar skin that is the result of an uninterrupted cycle of itching and scratching. The more that you itch, the more you will scratch, which in turn induces more itching. The hallmark of therapy is to break this cycle, which can be difficult, as scratching may occur in sleep. Topical steroids are among the treatments used. Some patients require an oral medication to help the itching and to help them not scratch in their sleep.

Cysts of the Vulva

A variety of benign cysts can affect the vulva. Sometimes no intervention is needed; however, a minor surgical procedure may be performed in some cases if the cyst is bothersome or diagnosis is uncertain.

Bartholin's Duct Cyst and Abscess

The Bartholin's glands are paired glands at the 4- and 8-o'clock positions at the vaginal opening. They produce a mucinous fluid that contributes to sexual lubrication. If the duct opening that opens out onto the vulva becomes blocked, fluid collects, and a cyst can form. The result is usually a painless, swollen fluid-filled cyst that generally feels like a lump. Sometimes this fluid can become infected, and then a small pocket of pus surrounded by inflamed tissue (also called an abscess) is the result. A Bartholin's abscess can be painful, but these abscesses are easily treated. A Bartholin's abscess is sometimes, but not always, secondary to gonorrhea. The cysts are painless but can be an annoyance. Treatment depends on the size of the cyst, if an infection is present, and how much discomfort the patient has. If the cyst is small and not infected, it can be treated at home with close observation and warm compresses. If it is infected and the patient is uncomfortable, the abscess may be drained (usually in the office), and sometimes antibiotics are necessary. Treatment of both cysts and abscesses may involve a minor surgical procedure. If the cyst has not become infected, a **marsupialization** is usually performed, in which a new opening to the duct is created. With an abscess, drainage is generally required.

Marsupialization

Refers to the surgical alteration of a cyst by making an incision and suturing the flaps to the adjacent tissue, creating an opening for the cyst to drain.

Epidermal Inclusion Cyst

Epidermal inclusions cysts are common on the vulva and may occur after invagination of the lining of the vulva after an episiotomy (the cut made during childbirth to widen the opening and allow the child's head to be delivered) or may occur spontaneously. They can be single or multiple and tend to increase with age. They cause no problems in most cases unless they become irritated or rupture, and thus, they only need to be removed if they annoy you in most cases. They have a "cheesy" material inside, composed of keratin, the acellular material on top of skin.

Benign Tumor-Like Lesions

A variety of benign conditions may present with a lump or bump and raise concern of a tumor.

Vestibular Adenosis

Adenosis is the persistence of glandular tissue in an area where it is normally lined by the kind of tissue you have in your mouth and vagina, squamous mucosa. It can be seen in women whose mothers took diethylstilbestrol during pregnancy, but may occur on its own. Women who are diethylstilbestrol daughters are usually under the care of providers who are familiar with the issues specific to the condition. For more information, see *http://www.cdc.gov/DES/consumers/.*

Adenosis

The persistence of glands in the vagina that are usually covered over by the vaginal squamous lining in the fetal life.

Endometriosis is the presence of endometrial tissue in an incorrect location. Sometimes endometrial tissue becomes implanted in the wrong place, often in areas of the pelvis.

Endometriosis

Endometriosis is the presence of endometrial tissue in an incorrect location. Endometrial tissue is normally found lining the uterus (womb) and is shed every month. When pregnancy doesn't occur in a reproductive aged woman, she has menstrual flow. Sometimes endometrial tissue becomes implanted in the wrong place, often in areas of the pelvis. The reason is unknown. Theories include that the endometrial tissue spreads by either blood vessels or lymphatic vessels or that it becomes attached to the wrong surfaces after backward menstruation out of the fallopian tubes or that one type of tissue simply turns into another. Probably most women experience some backward flow of their menses, and they don't all have endometriosis; thus, there must be some other or additional cause. The answer is not known. Endometriosis on the vulva most often occurs at the site of an episiotomy scar. Blue-black nodules may be seen, and these may swell, cause pain, or bleed at the time of menses because they cycle with the menstrual cycle.

Fibroepithelial Polyp (Acrochordon)

Fibroepithelial polyps

Refers to a benign polyp which is a projecting growth from a mucous skin surface.

Fibroepithelial polyps are simply skin tags. You can have them removed, but they will cause no trouble unless they get irritated.

Micropapillomatosis Labialis

Micropapillomatosis labialis

Small bumps on the labia minora which are a normal variant and do not represent an infection.

Some women have **micropapillomatosis labialis**, which looks almost like a carpet of little finger-like bumps in their vestibule. They are evenly spaced and look almost like the bristles of a rubber or plastic brush. They cause no trouble and need no therapy. They are merely an anatomic variant. It was originally thought that they might represent a form of genital warts, but this was shown to not be true (Figure 3).

Benign Neoplasms

The term neoplasm actually means "new growth," and they can be benign or malignant (cancerous). Benign neoplasms may need to be removed to rule out a malignancy when the diagnosis is not certain or for the comfort of the patient (Table 7).

Malignant Neoplasms

Although the most common malignancies of the vulva are those relating to HPV, a variety of other malignancies may rarely affect the vulva. Preinvasive (in situ) neoplasms have not yet broken through the basement membrane and have no ability to metastasize. Treating them is the best possible measure for preventing them from going on to become an invasive neoplasm, which can metastasize (Tables 8 and 9).

PART FIVE

Skin Disorders of the Vulva

I am scratching a lot, and my doctor says I have lichen simplex chronicus. What is that?

My doctor wants to do a vulvar biopsy. What should I expect?

Does lichen planus cause cancer?

More . . .

50. I am scratching a lot, and my doctor says I have lichen simplex chronicus. What is that?

Another name for lichen simplex chronicus is "neurodermatitis." People with eczema are more prone to this condition. This skin condition can affect the vulva (typically the hair-bearing labia majora and mons pubis), and it is characterized by chronic itching and the seemingly constant urge to scratch. The more you itch, the more you scratch, and the more you scratch, the more you itch. Patients fall into an "itch-scratch" cycle, and some even scratch in their sleep. The need to scratch occurs more commonly during periods of inactivity such as at bedtime. Emotional stress can provoke the itch, which is relieved temporarily by scratching. Some women feel inhibited going out in public for fear that they will need to scratch. Over time, the skin may become very thick and sometimes discolored. For the pathologist who may receive a biopsy from a patient with lichen simplex chronicus, a descriptive diagnosis of the findings, rather than a titled diagnosis may be given, or you may see a report that says "squamous cell hyperplasia."

51. How is lichen simplex chronicus treated?

Oral and topical medications are successfully used to treat lichen simplex chronicus.

Treatment depends on what is causing the itching. For example, underlying skin conditions such as lichen sclerosus can be associated with lichen simplex chronicus, and then treatment would be aimed at that primary condition. If no underlying condition is found, treatment is aimed at the lichen simplex chronicus directly. Oral and topical medications are successfully used to treat lichen simplex chronicus. Some patients may require a light sedative at night to help them from scratching in their sleep, and a cold compress (e.g., a cold bag of peas) can provide symptomatic relief. It usually takes several months before the skin appears normal again. Lichen simplex chronicus is not contagious.

52. *Does lichen simplex chronicus cause cancer?*

Lichen simple chronicus has not been shown to cause cancer or any other long-term or serious condition; however, some other dermatologic conditions that are associated with lichen simplex chronicus may have an increased risk of cancer. An example would be lichen sclerosus. Lichen sclerosus has been found in association with vulvar cancer in older women. It is not known whether lichen sclerosus is a risk factor for the development of vulvar cancer or whether it is just a coincidence.

53. *My doctor wants to do a vulvar biopsy. What should I expect?*

Doctors who specialize in vulvar disease are taught to biopsy liberally, as this often provides the most reliable diagnosis. The tissue needs to be looked at under a microscope so that a definitive diagnosis can be made. Your doctor may want you to stop aspirin or related medications before the biopsy in order to reduce bleeding. Be sure to ask before you make any changes in your medications.

First, you will receive numbing medicine in the area that is to be biopsied, similar to what is given in a dentist's office. Because only a tiny piece of skin is usually removed with a biopsy, a small amount is usually sufficient, and it is given in a very thin needle. You will feel a tiny stick and then a bit of burning when the numbing medicine goes in. After waiting until the area is numb, a small round blade, known as a "punch biopsy," or sometimes a scalpel blade, is used to remove the tiny piece of skin. Most punch biopsies are only 3 to 4 millimeters across, about a tenth of an inch! Sometimes, a stitch is placed where the biopsy was taken. You won't feel any of this. That's it!

You may be sore for a few days in the area, but this discomfort should be easily managed with acetaminophen. The area should be kept clean with mild soap and warm water. Your doctor will give you any special instructions. The removed tissue is placed in a preservative and is sent to a pathologist (a specialist physician who is able to look at biopsies under the microscope). It takes about a week to get the final results.

54. What does the pathologist do with my biopsy?

When a biopsy is performed, your provider places it in a jar of preservative and sends it to the pathology laboratory. Then the tissue undergoes a number of dehydrating steps that result in its preservation. Next, it is embedded in paraffin, creating a **paraffin block** (**Figure 4a–c**). The paraffin block is placed on a special machine called a **microtome**, where extremely thin slices (about 4.5 microns or about 0.0002 inches) are cut from this block. It is then placed on glass slides and stained and covered with a thin piece of glass called a coverslip. The slides are read by the pathologist, and a written report is sent to your provider. Multiple slides can be prepared from a single tissue block. This is sometimes helpful to

Paraffin block

A wax block. The biopsy is placed in the paraffin block so that thin slices of the biopsy can be made.

Microtome

An instrument for cutting very thin sections, as of organic tissue, for microscopic examination.

the pathologist if he or she wants to look at a deeper level of tissue or needs to evaluate any special stains. Also, duplicate slides can be prepared in case you are in need of a second opinion. This is true of any surgical

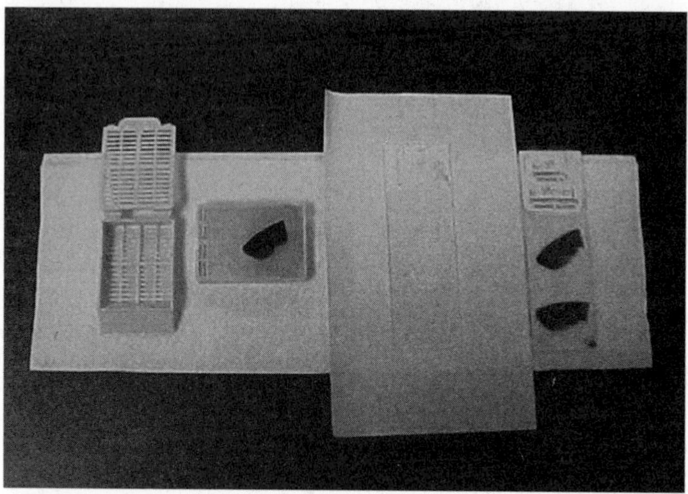

Figure 4a The pathologist places tissue in a plastic tissue cassette, where it is embedded in paraffin after dehydration. This paraffin block is used to cut an unstained slide (on paper) which is stained for reading under the microscope.

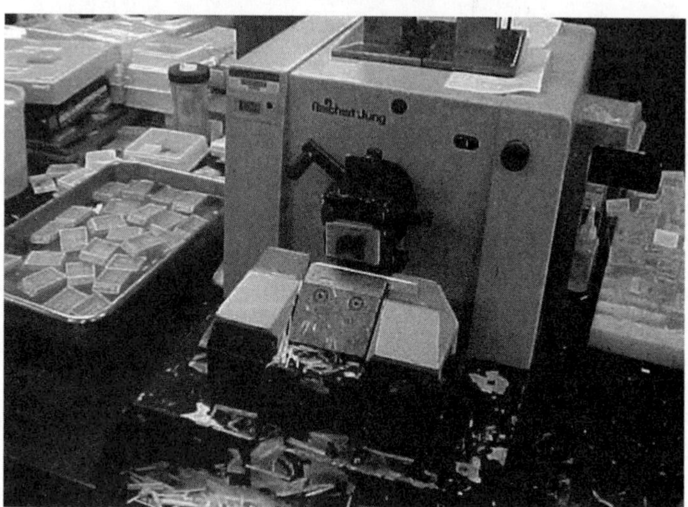

Figure 4b The unstained tissue sections are cut on a microtome.

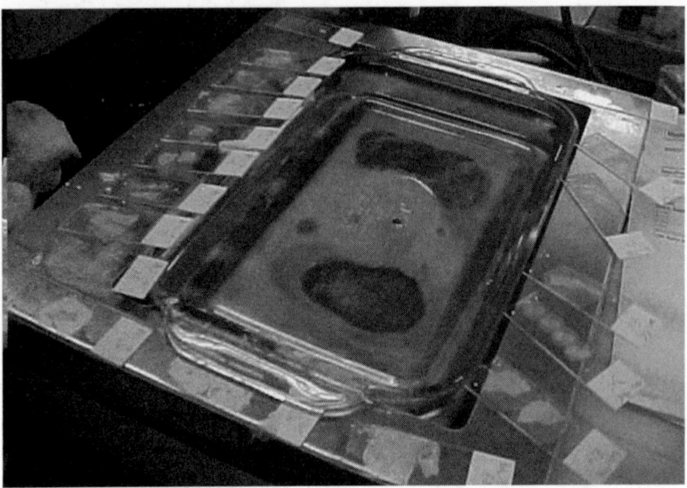

Figure 4c After cutting, the unstained sections are floated on a water bath and picked up onto slides for staining.

procedure you undergo. Pathology laboratories can provide a consultant of your choice duplicates of your slides for evaluation if you need it. There is usually paperwork that you will need to fill out.

55. *What is lichen sclerosus?*

Lichen sclerosus may be found on other areas of the body, but it is most common in the genital area.

Lichen sclerosus is a condition of the vulvar and perianal (surrounding the anus) skin. It causes white patches and thinning of the skin. It can be seen in women of all ages, as well as young girls, and it appears to be hereditary. Lichen sclerosus may be found on other areas of the body, but it is most common in the genital area. This condition may eventually lead to narrowing of the vaginal opening, with alteration of the appearance of the vulva. The labia minora may disappear, the clitoris may become buried, and the opening to the vagina (called the introitus) may become smaller, interfering with intercourse; however, treatment with a prescription-strength steroid, although not a cure, can help minimize the complications. Lichen sclerosus does not occur inside the vagina. Patients with lichen sclerosus typically describe itchiness or notice that things look "different"; however, they are sometimes asymptomatic. The cause of lichen sclerosus is unknown, although many clinicians feel that this is an autoimmune disease and it seems to be slightly more common in women with thyroid conditions. Lichen sclerosus may be definitively diagnosed with a vulvar biopsy.

Nina's comments:

I had vulvar itching and a dryness for years after I went through menopause. Intercourse was uncomfortable despite the fact that we used lubrication. I didn't think much of it because many of my friends said that was normal. Last year, my gynecologist said that the vulvar skin was turning white. She did a biopsy, and as it turned out, I have lichen sclerosus. She put me on a potent steroid cream, and after a few weeks, I began to feel better. She tapered me off the cream over the next several weeks, and now I apply it once a week for maintenance therapy. Because there is a small increased risk of vulvar cancer in women who have lichen sclerosus, I have a careful gynecologic examination every year. Also, because there is some association of lichen sclerosus with thyroid disease, my general doctor periodically checks my thyroid levels. This condition now hardly affects me—I just have to remember to apply the cream once a week!

56. How is lichen sclerosus treated?

Lichen sclerosus should be treated with a prescription-strength topical steroid cream. Typically, patients are asked to apply the cream once or twice a day. The frequency of the application is decreased with time until patients are on a maintenance dose, which may be applied, for example, once a week. Your provider will supply a specific schedule.

Lichen sclerosus is a chronic condition, meaning that it never goes away; however, with appropriate treatment, this disease can usually be easily managed with minimal impact on quality of life. If you have lichen sclerosus, a careful inspection of the vulva should be performed, along with your yearly gynecologic examination, and your health care provider should consider evaluating your thyroid.

57. Does lichen sclerosus cause cancer?

Lichen sclerosus may be associated with a low risk of vulvar cancer. Lichen sclerosus has been found in association with squamous cell carcinoma in older women. It is unknown whether the two conditions are related or are coincidental. Although large-scale studies have not been performed, it seems that appropriate treatment of lichen sclerosus decreases this slightly increased risk; therefore, seek treatment and have yearly vulvar examinations to catch problems early.

58. What is lichen planus?

Lichen planus is a rare inflammatory, noninfectious, noncontagious skin disorder that is found in many areas of the body, including the genitalia and mouth.

Lichen planus is a rare inflammatory, noninfectious, noncontagious skin disorder that is found in many areas of the body, including the genitalia and mouth. It usually causes soreness, rawness, and pain, especially with intercourse and/or itching, and the skin can be purplish in color, sometimes with bumps. Sometimes genital ulcerations are seen. There may be a lacy white pattern with areas of purple or red underneath or next to it when it involves the mouth or vagina. Scarring can occur, such as loss of the normal appearance of the vulva, with loss of the labia minora, and burying of the clitoris (also called clitoral phimosis). This may cause confusion with lichen sclerosus; however, unlike lichen sclerosus, which does not occur in the vagina, lichen planus may involve the vagina and with advanced disease can cause significant scarring of the vagina, with narrowing of the opening. A yellow discharge may be present. Lichen planus can be a bit more challenging to treat than lichen sclerosus and the cause of lichen planus is unknown. Your doctor may perform a biopsy to establish the diagnosis.

59. How is lichen planus treated?

As with other vulvar conditions, basic care, such as avoidance of products that can cause irritation and the use of a mild or no soap, should be instituted. Although lichen sclerosus is almost always treated with topical steroids, lichen planus also often requires oral steroids or other medications for adequate treatment, although sometimes intravaginal steroids are sufficient. Additionally, sometimes scarring that may occur in the vagina is best managed with dilators or very occasionally surgery. Lichen planus is a long-term condition and requires prolonged treatment and follow-up.

60. Does lichen planus cause cancer?

Rarely, lichen planus has been associated with squamous cell cancer of the vulva. The risk is considered to be about 2%; therefore, because lichen planus is a chronic condition that is not curable but can be managed, it is important to have regular exams with your health care provider. Lichen planus can have a significant impact on a woman's quality of life. Sometimes patients may see a gynecologist for their vulvar lichen planus and a dermatologist or internist for their oral disease.

PART SIX

Preinvasive Conditions and Vulvar Cancer

What are signs of vulvar cancer?

What is sentinel node sampling?

What is Paget's disease of the vulva?

More . . .

61. What is Vulvar Intraepithelial Neoplasia?

Vulvar Intraepithelial Neoplasia

A preinvasive carcinoma with no metastatic potential. The incidence of vulvar intraepithelial neoplasia has more than doubled in recent years, particularly in younger women.

VIN is becoming more common, probably because of the increasing occurrence of high-risk HPV infection that persists in younger women. Most cases of VIN occur in premenopausal women.

VIN stands for **Vulvar Intraepithelial Neoplasia**. VIN can be thought of as a precancerous condition of the vulva. An intraepithelial neoplasia is one that has not broken through the basement membrane, which is the structure at the bottom of the epithelial lining that limits the ability of a neoplasm to spread. Hence, an intraepithelial neoplasm is not capable of metastasizing. A high-risk type of HPV infection has been associated with both VIN and invasive vulvar cancer. The incidence of vulvar cancer is increasing, but at a slower rate than VIN. As previously discussed, a large percentage of women who become infected with HPV will clear detectible levels of the virus from their systems; however, if the high-risk types of the virus are persistent, the risk of VIN is increased. VIN is becoming more common, probably because of the increasing occurrence of high risk HPV infection that persists in younger women. Most cases of VIN occur in premenopausal women.

62. Who gets VIN?

Risk factors for VIN include persistent high-risk HPV infection, cigarette smoking, and immunodeficiency, including not only HIV, but other conditions associated with immune deficiency, or immunosuppression from illness or medication. Cigarette smoking alters the local immunity of the lower genital tract and makes HPV-related lesions of the vulva, vagina, and cervix harder to control. If you are a smoker and you are diagnosed with VIN or any other HPV-related lesion, stopping smoking is very helpful.

63. *How is VIN diagnosed?*

Up to 50% of patients with VIN are asymptomatic at the time of diagnosis. You may have no symptoms, or you may feel itching, burning, or pain in the vulva. Typically, the lesions of VIN have a raised surface, and about 25% are dark colored; the remainder might be pink, gray, red, or white. The lesions may be flat or raised and may be single or multiple. Because these symptoms can be caused by other conditions that are not precancerous, some women fail to recognize the seriousness of their condition and attempt to treat the problem themselves with over-the-counter remedies. Sometimes even doctors may not recognize the condition at first. The diagnosis is based on a careful inspection by a health care provider who specializes in vulvar disease and a biopsy of the affected area.

64. *What is vulvoscopy?*

To help diagnose abnormalities such as VIN, the vulva may be examined by **vulvoscopy**. During this procedure, a special microscope called a **colposcope** is usually used to examine the vulva. Vulvoscopy is a painless outpatient procedure. You will be asked to lie on your back with your legs in supports, just as if you were getting a Pap smear. Usually diluted acetic acid (vinegar) may be sprayed or painted on your vulva. This will allow any abnormal cells to become more visibly prominent. Although this is not painful, it may cause some mild irritation. The clinician may perform a biopsy (discussed previously here) during the vulvoscopy procedure. Vulvoscopy is not performed as commonly as **colposcopy**, which is the same instrument, but is used to examine the cervix after an abnormal Pap smear. Some providers examine the vulva with a hand-held magnifying glass.

Vulvoscopy

A special microscope is used to examine the vulva under high-power visualization. Vulvoscopy is a painless outpatient procedure.

Colposcope

A magnifying and photographic device used as an aid in the diagnostic examination of the female vulva, vagina, and cervix.

Colposcopy

A procedure where the cervix is visualized with a special microscope called a colposcope. It is a painless, outpatient procedure. Sometimes a biopsy is taken at the same time.

65. Will I need surgery?

Not necessarily. VIN can be readily treated and the most common treatment options include topical **chemotherapy**, carbon dioxide laser ablation, and surgical excision. Topical treatment may include 5-fluorouracil. The advantages of topical treatments include minimal scarring and avoidance of surgery; however, these treatments usually cause local irritation and are not always successful. Additionally, these treatments may not be as effective in hair-bearing areas. Some clinicians feel that topical treatments are only for women who cannot undergo other ablative or excisional treatments. Another topical treatment that has been used with mixed results is imiquimod, an immune modulator.

Chemotherapy
The treatment of disease by means of chemicals that have a specific toxic effect or that selectively destroy cancerous tissue.

VIN can be readily treated and the most common treatment options include topical chemotherapy, carbon dioxide laser ablation, and surgical excision.

Laser ablation is an effective option for non–hair-bearing areas. It is typically performed as an outpatient and does not require repeat applications by the patient. Disadvantages of this option are that it can be painful and take weeks to heal. Surgical removal of VIN in many instances may be the best therapy. There is immediate removal of the affected tissue, and healing is much faster than with the laser. For smaller lesions, this treatment can frequently be accomplished in the clinician's office and has the advantage of providing a tissue specimen for pathologic review (unlike the laser, which destroys tissue). This can be important in the uncommon case of an unsuspected invasive carcinoma next to the VIN lesion. The treatment option that is best for you depends on the type and location of the VIN, your overall health status, and the experience and comfort of your health care provider with the different treatment options. Regardless of which treatment option is used, early detection and treatment of VIN may prevent development of vulvar cancer. The risk of vulvar cancer developing from VIN increases with age, smoking, and immunosuppression.

Smoking cessation is the best thing you can do if you have VIN, in addition to following up with the treatment and posttreatment evaluations recommended by your health care provider.

66. *Will I need chemotherapy or radiation?*

Chemotherapy and **radiation** are treatments that are generally reserved for some invasive cancers. VIN is not typically treated with systemic chemotherapy or radiation. VIN may be treated with laser therapy in select patients.

Radiation
The treatment of disease (especially cancer) by exposure to a radioactive substance

67. *What does it mean to have vulvar cancer?*

Vulvar carcinoma (cancer) is the fourth most common female genital tract cancer and comprises 5% of malignancies of the female genital tract. Although the rate of invasive vulvar carcinoma has remained stable over the past 20 years, the incidence of VIN has more than doubled, particularly in younger women. Vulvar carcinoma is seen most commonly in postmenopausal women (unlike VIN). The average age at diagnosis of invasive vulvar cancer is 65 years. Most cases of vulvar cancer are caused by squamous cell carcinoma originating in the epidermis (the top layer of skin) of the vulva.

There are essentially two different "types" of vulvar cancer, those associated with HPV and those that are not.

There are essentially two different "types" of vulvar cancer, those associated with HPV and those that are not. The HPV-associated lesions occur in younger women, sometimes in their 40s and 50s. These cancers are associated more frequently with previous and co-existing VIN, and they have a better prognosis overall than the vulvar cancers not associated with HPV. The other kind of vulvar cancer, although it looks the same to the eye and under the microscope, is not associated with HPV. This is the one seen more often in women 65 years old and older. Overall, the prognosis is less favorable than in the HPV-related lesions, although if caught early, it can be cured. Non–HPV-related vulvar cancers may be associated with lichen sclerosus, but it is still not known whether lichen sclerosus is a risk factor. Non–HPV-related vulvar carcinoma may also be associated with a lesion called "differentiated VIN," a very uncommon form of VIN not associated with HPV. Differentiated VIN is thought to be of greater risk for progressing to non–HPV-related invasive vulvar squamous cell carcinoma than usual VIN is thought to be for progressing to HPV-related invasive squamous cell carcinoma of the vulva.

68. What are signs of vulvar cancer?

Most vulvar cancers are found on the labia majora. Typically, a lesion is present in the form of a lump or an ulcer. This lesion may be associated with no symptoms, but is often associated with itching, irritation and sometimes local bleeding and discharge. There may also be pain with urination and sexual activity. Most women with vulvar cancer present with itching and some kind of visible abnormality.

69. How is vulvar cancer diagnosed?

Early diagnosis of vulvar cancer requires maintenance of a high index of suspicion and biopsy of anything that looks abnormal on the vulva. Gynecologists and dermatologists with a special interest in the vulva are taught to biopsy the vulva liberally. A thorough gynecologic examination should always include a visual inspection of the external genitalia. In the case of a vulvar cancer, examination of the vulva may reveal abnormalities such as an ulcer, a mass, or even just a skin discoloration. In order to find out what the abnormality is, a biopsy should be performed. These can usually be performed in the office with local anesthesia, and the results usually take about a week to return from the laboratory.

At initial evaluation, a detailed physical examination should be performed that includes measurements of the vulvar lesion, assessment for extension to adjacent structures, bimanual pelvic examination, and assessment of inguinal lymph node involvement. Because cancers of the female genital tract can exist in multiple locations, the vagina and cervix should be carefully inspected, and a Pap smear of the cervix should be performed. Your provider may send you to get additional imaging studies.

70. Are there risk factors for vulvar cancer?

Risk factors for vulvar cancer include cigarette smoking, HPV-related conditions such as vulvar or cervical intraepithelial neoplasia, HPV infection, immunodeficiency syndromes (such as HIV), and a prior history of cervical cancer. For vulvar cancer not related to HPV, differentiated VIN is considered a risk factor. It is unclear whether lichen sclerosus increases the chances of developing vulvar cancer.

71. Is there anything I did to cause this?

Although there are known risk factors for vulvar cancer, probably other risk factors exist that we don't know about. Many women who have risk factors for vulvar cancer do not

Many women who have risk factors for vulvar cancer do not develop the disease, and thus, it is unlikely that you did any one specific thing that caused you to get the vulvar cancer.

develop the disease, and thus, it is unlikely that you did any one specific thing that caused you to get the vulvar cancer.

72. Is there any way to prevent vulvar cancer?

Prevention is the best medicine! Routine gynecologic examinations by a health care provider are an effective screening tool. Another way to minimize your chances of getting vulvar cancer is self-inspection. You can periodically inspect the vulvar region with a mirror. Any visible abnormalities can then be brought to the attention of your health care provider. Vulvar cancer can be prevented by avoiding known risk factors when possible, such as minimizing one's exposure to HPV through choosing partners wisely, using condoms, avoiding cigarette smoking, and having regular physical checkups as well as routine Pap smears and pelvic examinations. Treatment of preinvasive VIN lesions if they are found is also a good way to try to prevent vulvar cancer. If a cancer is present, early detection will maximize the chances of a cure.

73. Will I need surgery?

You will probably need some sort of surgical treatment for vulvar cancer. Surgery is typically the first-line therapy. Surgery used to include a much larger excision, which was associated with more complications; however, now surgical treatment is more tailored to the specific size and location of the tumor for the individual patient, and the excisions are often much more localized and smaller, particularly with early diagnosis. Radiation therapy and chemotherapy are usually not a first-choice treatment but may be used in selected cases.

74. What kind of surgery is done?

Surgery is one of the main treatments of vulvar cancer, and it is usually accomplished by a procedure called a **radical vulvectomy**. This includes removal of vulvar tissue as well as the lymph nodes from the groin. Depending on the location of the cancer and its size, lesser excisions may be possible. This is something that needs to be discussed with your gynecologic oncology surgeon. Potential complications of such surgery include wound infection, sexual problems, lower leg swelling, and blood clots in the legs. Surgery is significantly more extensive when vulvar cancer has spread to the urethra, vagina, and rectum. In cases of early vulvar carcinoma, the surgery may be less involved and disfiguring and may consist of removal of the vulva or a portion of the vulva only. Hence, it is very important to seek treatment as soon as possible.

Radical vulvectomy

A surgical procedure performed to treat vulvar cancer. It involves removal of vulvar tissue and is usually combined with resection of the lymph nodes from the groin.

75. What is sentinel node sampling?

Cancer usually spreads first to the **sentinel lymph nodes**. It is thought that if the sentinel lymph nodes are negative for cancer that any other regional lymph nodes will be negative too, as the sentinel node has to be "passed" first. By checking the sentinel node and getting a negative result, removal of additional lymph nodes can sometimes be avoided. This decreases the complications of lymph node excisions, including greater risk of infection, bleeding, and chronic swelling (**lymphedema**). Sentinel lymph node sampling is well established in the surgical treatment of malignant **melanomas** of the skin and in breast cancer surgery. It is being investigated in a variety of other cancer surgical procedures, including in the treatment of vulvar cancer. Removing and examining only one or two sentinel nodes in the groin and upper leg (as opposed to many

Sentinel lymph nodes

The first lymph nodes a cancer usually spreads to.

Lymphedema

The accumulation of lymph in soft tissue with accompanying swelling, often of the extremities, sometimes caused by inflammation, obstruction, or removal of lymph channels.

Melanoma

Any of several types of skin tumors characterized by the malignant growth of melanocytes (pigment forming skin cells).

lymph nodes, as used to be the standard of care) have been shown to be effective in detecting whether cancer has spread in women with early-stage vulvar cancer. Additionally, this technique results in fewer negative side effects compared with the standard approach of removing many lymph nodes. The surgeon must have extensive experience in performing sentinel lymph node dissections, and the pathology laboratory should be informed that the nodes submitted are sentinel nodes so that special stains can be done in order to prevent very small **metastases** from being overlooked. Identification of the sentinel node for the surgeon is achieved by injection at a marker that goes to that node first. The marker can be a radioactive material that can be detected with a radiation detector, a blue dye visible to the naked eye, or a combination.

The stage of your vulvar cancer, what type of surgery and other treatment you have had, as well as your overall physical and mental health will dictate when you may resume sexual relationships.

Metastases

The transference of malignant or cancerous cells to other parts of the body by way of the blood or lymphatic vessels or membranous surfaces.

76. Can I ever have sex again?

The stage of your vulvar cancer (whether it has spread and if so how far), what type of surgery and other treatment you have had, as well as your overall physical and mental health will dictate when you may resume sexual relationships. Women with more advanced disease, including those who require vulvar reconstruction, will most likely take longer to heal than women who have had less radical surgery.

Sarah's comments:

I was diagnosed with vulvar cancer last year. After I was diagnosed, things happened so quickly. I had surgery a week after I was diagnosed, and I also had reconstructive work by a plastic surgeon all during the same operation. This team of doctors performed the surgery so that I was able to keep a sexually functional vagina.

I have to say that the recovery took a long time. I was very uncomfortable for the first week or so after the surgery; I took pain medication by mouth every few hours. The discomfort started to get better after the first week. In the second week, I got a skin infection in some of the stitches. I took antibiotics for that and had a wound care nurse come to my house every day to look at it and change the dressings. Even walking around was difficult at first.

Luckily, I did not need chemotherapy or radiation. I am a member of a support group, and I have met other women who are going through this or have been through it. This support group was a key component of my recovery process; it is comforting to know that I am not the only one who has been through this.

77. Will I need chemotherapy or radiation?

Some patients with vulvar cancer will not be best treated with surgery. Radiation therapy and chemotherapy are usually not a primary choice of therapy but may be used in selected cases of advanced vulvar cancer. This is something to discuss with your gynecologic **oncologist**.

Oncologist

A physician who specializes in the treatment of cancer.

78. What can I expect with chemotherapy?

Some patients with advanced vulvar cancer undergo preoperative radiation therapy, with or without concurrent chemotherapy. Any negative side effects that you experience depend on which chemotherapy is used. Some chemotherapeutic agents have more side effects than others. Preventive measures to avoid or minimize some of the unpleasant side effects have improved over the years. These concerns need to be discussed with your providers so that the answers you receive are specific to your own situation.

79. What can I expect with radiation?

Some patients undergo radiation therapy for vulvar cancer either before or after surgery. You will most likely have a consultation with a radiation oncologist, a doctor who specializes in radiation therapy. Depending on your overall health status and the stage and location of your disease, this will determine where the radiation will be and for how long.

80. What is the prognosis for vulvar cancer?

The prognosis of vulvar cancer depends on many things, including the stage of the cancer and the overall health status of the patient. For patients with vulvar squamous cell carcinomas, the spread or lack of spread of the cancer to the lymph nodes is the single most important prognostic factor. The prognosis of vulvar cancer shows overall about a 75% survival at 5 years. Five-year survival decreases to about 20% when pelvic lymph nodes are involved but is better than 90% in patients with stage I disease; therefore, early diagnosis is a must!

Staging

A standardized system of determining if a cancer has spread and how advanced a cancer is. It is different for each type of cancer.

81. What is staging?

The term **staging** refers to a standardized system of determining whether a cancer has spread and how advanced a cancer is. Every type of cancer has its own staging system; however, the staging system for each cancer is similar in structure. Usually a stage I tumor is confined to where it started from, and a stage IV tumor is widespread to other organs. Stages II and III are therefore in between. Treatment of cancers is based partly on the stage of a tumor. The stage also gives some information on how well a patient will do, based on outcomes of groups of patients with the same stage, although everyone is different and any one patient may have a tumor that behaves differently than expected. Staging of tumors may be assessed clinically in some cases (i.e., by examination and imaging studies or by how far the tumor is found to have spread at surgery by the pathology laboratory findings in other cases, or often as a combination of both). Staging is usually a combination of the tumor itself (T), the status of the lymph nodes (N), and whether there are metastases (M). The TNM score is then converted into stage I through stage IV. In the case of vulvar cancer, the stage depends on what is found at the time of surgery. Staging and treatment should be handled by an oncologist who is familiar with gynecologic cancers. Stage I describes the early stage of the cancer that still is confined to the site of origin. Stages II and III define less or more extensive extensions to adjacent tissue and lymph nodes, whereas stage IV indicates more widely metastatic disease.

Every type of cancer has its own staging system; however, the staging system for each cancer is similar in structure. Usually a stage I tumor is confined to where it started from, and a stage IV tumor is widespread. Stages II and III are therefore in between.

Staging of any cancer is given at the time of the definitive initial therapy. If a tumor recurs or spreads later, the stage is not changed, as this would not allow for meaningful statistics to be evaluated on tumor outcomes. It is used predominantly for prognosis and treatment planning. For any specific cancer, studies will have indicated the expected range of outcomes for a given stage, expressed as 5-year survival or as disease-free interval; however, with newer therapies coming out all the time, outcomes are always improving. The staging for vulvar cancer according to the International Federation of Gynecology & Obstetrics is shown here. Tis is the same as VIN, a preinvasive carcinoma with no metastatic potential.

Tumor (T)

Tis: The cancer is not invading into the underlying tissues.

T1: The cancer is growing only in the vulva or perineum and is smaller than 2 cm (about 0.8 inches).

- **T1a**: The cancer invades no more than 1 mm into underlying tissue.
- **T1b**: The cancer invades more than 1 mm into underlying tissue.

T2: The cancer is growing only in the vulva or perineum and is larger than 2 cm (about 0.8 inches).

T3: The cancer is growing into the lower urethra, anus, or vagina.

T4: The cancer is growing into the upper urethra, bladder, or rectum or into the pubic bone.

Lymph Node Spread (N)

N0: No lymph node spread.

N1: Spread to lymph nodes on the same side as the cancerous vulva

N2: Spread to lymph nodes on the same and opposite side as the cancerous vulva

Distant Spread (M)

M0: No distant spread

M1: Spread to distant sites.

Stage Grouping

The grouping of T, N, and M determines the stage.

Stage 0: Tis, N0, M0: This is a very early cancer found in the surface of the skin of the vulva only. Stage 0 squamous cell cancer of the vulva is also known as carcinoma in situ.

Stage I: T1, N0, M0: The cancer is in the vulva or the perineum or both. The tumor is 2 cm or less (about 0.8 inch) in diameter and has not spread to lymph nodes or distant sites.

- *Stage IA:* T1a: Stage I cancers with invasion no deeper than 1 mm (about 1⁄25 inch).
- *Stage IB:* T1b: Stage I cancers that have invaded deeper than 1 mm.

Stage II: T2, N0, M0: The cancer is in the vulva or perineum or both, and the tumor is larger than 2 cm. It has not spread to lymph nodes or distant sites.

Stage III: T1-T2, N1, M0, or T3, N0-N1, M0: Cancer is found in the vulva or perineum or both or has spread to nearby tissues, such as the urethra, vagina, or anus, and/or has spread to nearby lymph nodes on one side of the groin. It has not spread to distant sites.

Stage IVA: T1–3, N2, M0, or T4, N0-N2, M0: Cancer has spread to lymph nodes on both sides of the groin, or it has spread beyond nearby tissues to the upper part of the urethra, bladder, rectum, or pelvic bone.

Stage IVB: Cancer has spread to distant organs of the body. This is the most advanced stage of cancer.

Recurrent: The cancer has come back after treatment.

82. How does vulvar cancer spread?

Local extension

Spread from an organ or tissue to an adjacent one.

Cancers can spread by **local extension**, as well as by getting into the blood circulation or the lymphatic circulation. Vulvar squamous cell cancers tend to spread via the local lymphatic system. The cancer cells travel in the lymph system from the labia majora to the upper vulva and mons pubis and then to the lymph nodes of the groin. The deepest lymph node in the groin is called the Cloquet's node, and tumor cells that travel beyond this node can enter the lymph nodes of the pelvis. Vulvar cancer can also invade the vagina, urethra, and rectum by local extension.

Cancers can spread by local extension, as well as by getting into the blood circulation or the lymphatic circulation.

83. What happens if vulvar cancer comes back after therapy?

Close follow-up after being treated for vulvar cancer is a must, just as for any other cancer. Recurrences are most commonly seen in the first 2 years after treatment but have been seen up to several years after treatment. If you feel that you have a recurrence, go to your doctor immediately for an evaluation. If you have a recurrence of your disease, you will need to be evaluated to see how extensive the recurrence is, and then treatment can be specifically tailored to your individual situation.

84. How do I know whether I am "cured"?

After completing treatment for vulvar cancer, patients should be followed very closely. One follow-up plan is to be seen every 3 to 4 months for 2 years and then every 6 months for the next 3 years, and then annually, but your provider will give you a specific schedule. In addition to examination of the vulva and groin, a pelvic examination and a rectal examination should be performed at each visit. Pap smears of the cervix or vagina should also be performed at appropriate intervals. Although there are rare late recurrences, after the 5-year mark has been passed, it is more likely than not that you are free of cancer.

85. Does vulvar cancer cause pain?

Vulvar cancer in its early stages is not usually associated with pain. As the cancer spreads, there may be discomfort in the pelvic area. The signs and symptoms of early invasive vulvar cancer are similar to those of symptomatic VIN. As the tumor grows, a distinct looking mass or ulceration is more likely to be seen. The most common sign is a red, pink, or white bump or bumps with a wart-like or raw surface. About half of the women with vulvar cancer complain of persistent itching as well as a growth. Some also complain of pain, burning, painful urination, bleeding, and discharge not associated with the normal menstrual period (in cycling women). A painless ulcer that persists for more than a month is another sign. Knowing what to look for can sometimes help with early detection, but it is even better not to wait until you notice symptoms. Have regular Pap tests and pelvic examinations!

86. What are the different types of vulvar cancer?

Squamous cell carcinoma is the most common type of vulvar cancer (as discussed previously here). Other less common types include malignant melanoma, invasive **Paget's disease**, a Bartholin gland cancer, and a verrucous carcinoma.

Paget's disease

Presents with a very itchy, rashy-looking, red, oozy area on the vulva. It can be thought of a cancer that spreads very slowly; however, it can be associated with adenocarcinomas (cancer of a gland) elsewhere in the body.

The appearance of a darkly pigmented growth or a change in a mole that has been present for years may indicate a vulvar melanoma. Unlike melanomas that occur on the body, vulvar melanomas are not associated with sun exposure, and it is not known why they occur in this region. Although vulvar cancer in general is rare, melanoma of the vulva is the second most common type of vulvar cancer, comprising about 10% of the cases. The *ABCD* rule used to evaluate skin lesions can help to distinguish a noncancerous mole from one that could be melanoma; however, some melanomas do not fit the ABCD rule.

Asymmetry: One-half of the mole does not match the other.

Border irregularity: The edges of the mole are ragged or notched.

Color: The color over the mole is not the same. There may be differing shades of tan, brown, or black and sometimes patches of red, blue, or white.

Diameter: The mole is wider than 6 mm (about ¼ inch).

The most important sign of melanoma is a change in size, shape, or color of a mole. Melanoma of the vulva is a very aggressive condition, usually because it is not caught early enough. Providers know to have a low threshold to biopsy pigmented lesions. Melanoma of the vulva is staged differently than squamous cell carcinoma, using a modification of the staging used for skin melanoma, but taking into account the unique geography of the vulvar skin.

Bartholin's Gland Cancer

The Bartholin glands are located at 4- and 8-o'clock at the opening of the vagina. These glands are important for vaginal lubrication. A distinct mass on either side of the opening of the vagina may indicate a cancer of a Bartholin gland, particularly in a woman over the age of 40 years, although these cancers are very rare. Similar symptoms may be due to a Bartholin gland cyst, which is much more common. If you are older than 40 years, your provider may take a biopsy of the gland at the time of surgical intervention.

Soreness, itchiness, and a red, scaly area are symptoms of Paget's disease of the vulva. Paget's disease is usually an in situ carcinoma of specialized type, although it can rarely become invasive (discussed later here).

A verrucous carcinoma is the one subtype of invasive squamous cell vulvar cancer that has a particularly good prognosis. It appears as cauliflower-like growths similar to genital warts, but much larger. They are probably caused by a specific type of HPV. These too are uncommon. They can get quite large and can recur on the vulva but almost never spread to the lymph nodes in the groin.

87. What is Paget's disease of the vulva?

Patients with vulvar Paget's disease generally present with a very itchy, rashy-looking, red, oozy area on the vulva. This disease typically occurs in older, postmenopausal white women. It is not unusual for vulvar Paget's disease to be misdiagnosed as eczema or contact dermatitis because of its eczema-like appearance. Approximately 15% to 20% of women with vulvar Paget's

Patients with vulvar Paget's disease generally present with a very itchy, rashy-looking, red, oozy area on the vulva. This disease typically occurs in older, postmenopausal white women.

Adenocarcinoma

A malignant tumor of a gland-like structure

disease have an underlying other type of cancer called an **adenocarcinoma**. Adenocarcinomas arise from glandular tissue. If an underlying adenocarcinoma in association with Paget's disease is present, it may arise from the sweat glands within the vulvar skin. Also, about 20% to 30% of patients with vulvar Paget's disease will have or will go on to develop an adenocarcinoma elsewhere in the body. The most commonly observed sites are breast, colon, rectum, and the upper female genital tract. Because of this, if you are diagnosed with Paget's disease, your health care provider should check you for these possibilities.

88. How is Paget's disease of the vulva diagnosed?

In order to confirm Paget's disease of the vulva, the clinician will most often do a biopsy of the itchy, red area. Under a microscope, specific Paget's cells recognizable to the pathologist are seen within the epithelium. Paget's disease is usually considered a form of carcinoma in situ. It hasn't broken through the basement membrane, a structure that is the bottom-most part of the epithelium and therefore can't spread to other parts of the body. Rarely, Paget's disease does break through the basement membrane, and then it is called invasive Paget's disease. Paget's disease, even though it is usually not invasive, is often associated with other invasive cancers, and you will need to be evaluated for these (see Question 87).

89. How is Paget's disease of the vulva treated?

Surgery is the most common way to treat Paget's disease of the vulva. This is done with a wide local excision—the standard treatment for vulvar Paget's disease. The idea is to excise all of the disease with a sufficient rim (margin) of normal tissue. The underlying dermis (deep skin) should be removed for adequate microscopic evaluation. This is because vulvar Paget's disease usually extends far beyond the red eczema-like–appearing abnormality that is seen with the naked eye. Your surgeon may make sure that enough is removed by asking the pathologist to perform an intraoperative consultation, called a frozen section. The tissue to be evaluated, here the edges of the proposed excision, can be looked at right away by the pathologist. The pathology laboratory prepares a slide immediately by freezing the tissue while you are having the surgery. The pathologist can then look at it while you are having surgery, and if the area is not normal, more tissue can be excised then and there. A frozen section slide is different from the usual way tissue is made into slides, which takes longer (hours or overnight) but provides a better quality slide. Frozen-section diagnosis (where the removed tissue is examined right away by a pathologist) of the surgical margins while still in the operating room is often performed to ensure complete removal of the Paget's disease.

90. Is there a relationship between vulvar cancer and hormone replacement therapy?

No well-documented relationship exists between vulvar squamous cell cancer and hormone replacement therapy; however, given that this is a malignancy that can be associated with HPV and other genital tract cancers, your provider should get a full medical history.

91. What type of doctor treats vulvar cancer? What type of doctor treats other benign diseases of the vulva?

Gynecologic oncologists are doctors who have had extra medical training and are specially trained to diagnose and treat cancers of the female genital tract (ovarian, cervical, vaginal, uterine, and vulvar cancer). They have advanced training in surgical therapies for these conditions. Some of them may also administer chemotherapy, but you may be referred to a medical oncologist, an internist with advanced training in chemotherapeutic cancer treatments. Radiation is administered by doctors called radiation oncologists. In any condition requiring a team of specialists, such as cancer, it is important that all of the specialties communicate with each other, and you should be aware of which physician is serving as the "captain of the ship." Be informed, and participate in your care!

Benign (noncancerous) conditions of the vulva may be seen and treated by any gynecologist; however, as medical advances are made and we learn more about the female genital tract and vulva, some gynecologists have become subspecialized and have developed a special interest in the vulva and are considered as "vulvologists." Many of the conditions affecting the vulva are uniquely dermatologic; thus, some dermatologists have a special interest in the region, and they are also vulvologists. They may also be more attuned to a melanoma because of their experience. A variety of healthcare professionals also have specialized training and interest, and physical therapists, sexual medicine doctors, and advanced practice nurses among others may be able to help you with a vulvar condition. The most prominent vulvar specialists in the world are members of the International Society for the Study of Vulvovaginal Diseases. This organization has a website at *http://www.ISSVD.org* that has information for patients as well as health care providers.

92. Can other types of vulvar conditions turn into cancer?

Yes. The two conditions most commonly associated with vulvar cancer are VIN and lichen sclerosus. VIN can progress to squamous cell carcinoma of the vulva, although this is less likely to happen than with the precancerous lesions of the cervix progressing to frank cervical cancer. Older age, smoking, and immunosuppression increase the risk of progression. Lichen sclerosus, described previously, is often associated with the non–HPV-related squamous cell carcinomas of the vulva found in older women. Whether it is causative or just associated is not clear. Lichen sclerosus is a skin disorder that may also affect the vulva. It is characterized by a thinning and whitening of the skin, as well as itchiness. Women with lichen sclerosus have a 3% to 5% chance of developing vulvar cancer over the course of their lifetime. Lichen sclerosus should be thought of as a manageable chronic condition of the vulva. Women with lichen sclerosus should see their provider for a vulvar examination at recommended intervals.

The two conditions most commonly associated with vulvar cancer are VIN and lichen sclerosus.

93. Is my daughter or other family members at risk of developing vulvar cancer if I have it?

Many cancers have a familial predisposition, but no strong familial predisposition to vulvar cancer has been found. Nevertheless, all women, regardless of family history, should have routine gynecologic examinations.

94. If I have had a sexually transmitted disease, am I at increased risk for vulvar cancer?

Many different sexually transmitted diseases exist, and they can have a variety of long-term effects. Currently, it seems that many sexually transmitted diseases as well as nonspecific vaginitis are not associated with vulvar cancer. There *may* be a slightly increased risk with a subset of sexually transmitted diseases, including herpes simplex virus 2, although this is not known for certain. There is a higher risk with HPV infection of the lower genital tract. Although most vulvar cancers occur in women older than 55 years of age, those that occur in younger women are frequently associated with HPV. Also, it takes years (maybe even decades) for vulvar cancer to develop after being infected with HPV.

Routine Pap smears and physical examinations are an effective way to screen for cervical and vulvar cancers. Regular gynecological exams are necessary to detect precancerous conditions (called vulvar intraepithelial neoplasia) that can *easily* be treated before the cancer becomes invasive. Performing proper genital hygiene to prevent infection and inflammation and not engaging in risky sexual behavior may reduce the risk of vulvar cancer.

Because some vulvar cancers are a form of skin cancer, the American Cancer Society recommends self-examination of the vulva with a mirror. Your health care provider should evaluate any new moles or growths.

PART SEVEN

Pregnancy and Menopause

Ever since I went through menopause, the vulvar area is more sensitive. Why?

I am pregnant. Do I have any additional concerns relating to the vulva or vagina?

I am menopausal. Do I still need to see a gynecologist? I have had a hysterectomy. Do I still need a gynecologist?

More . . .

95. I have gone through menopause. Is it possible for the vulva as well as the vagina to become dry?

Many young women who have been on oral contraceptive pills (and therefore have altered hormone levels), as well as women who have gone through menopause, may experience atrophic vestibulitis, meaning that their vulva has become irritated and sensitive because of a loss of hormonal protection and stimulation.

Yes! The vulva is also *very* sensitive to female hormones, just like the vagina. In fact, recent evidence indicates that the female vulva has even more testosterone receptors than estrogen receptors. Interestingly, many young women who have been on oral contraceptive pills (and therefore have altered hormone levels), as well as women who have gone through menopause, may experience atrophic vestibulitis, meaning that their vulva has become irritated and sensitive because of a loss of hormonal protection and stimulation. Women who have gone through menopause frequently report vaginal dryness, but they are probably also experiencing vulvar dryness as well, which can be just as irritating, if not more so. If this is a problem, discuss it with your provider, and see whether some topical estrogen therapy is a safe and useful therapy for you.

96. Ever since I went through menopause, the vulvar area is more sensitive. Why?

Female hormones such as progesterone and especially estrogen help to keep the female genitals healthy. Estrogen helps to maintain the blood supply to the vulva and vagina, thus helping to ensure good health in these areas. At the time of menopause when estrogen levels decrease, a variety of changes may occur, including thinning of the vulvar skin. The vulvar skin is sensitive to the effects of estrogen and without it becomes delicate, thin, dry, and sometimes more sensitive.

97. I am pregnant. Do I have any additional concerns relating to the vulva or vagina?

In general, no additional measures, other than routine basic hygiene, need to be taken to care for the genitalia during pregnancy. Sometimes during pregnancy, the vulva can become darker or turn a purplish color. This is due to varicose veins, which commonly occur on the legs and thighs but may also occur in the vulva or vagina, especially during late pregnancy. This occurs because women retain a lot of weight and fluid during pregnancy and the fetus may compress some parts of the pelvis, causing engorgement of the veins in the vulva/vagina. Varicose veins on the vulva/vagina typically resolve after delivery. Toward the end of pregnancy, as the baby grows and becomes heavier, you may feel vaginal pressure. Some women may feel as if their vagina is more sensitive. Toward full term, you may notice a thick discharge that is sometimes blood tinged. This is known as a mucus plug and is an indication that you may go into labor very soon!

98. Sometimes I feel as if there is a bulge in my vagina, what could this be?

Many women as they get older experience pelvic organ prolapse, sometimes called "pelvic relaxation," particularly if they have delivered children vaginally. Pelvic organ prolapse is defined as the descent of one or all of the female pelvic organs: the bladder, uterus, vagina, and rectum. This condition is more common as women get older, but it may occur in women in their twenties and thirties. No one knows exactly what causes pelvic organ prolapse; however, known risk factors include multiple vaginal deliveries, chronic coughing, chronic straining to have a bowel movement, and there seems to be some hereditary predisposition. Obesity is also a risk factor. Some of these risk factors are related to increased pressure inside the abdomen. Typically, women with pelvic organ prolapse will feel a "bulge" coming out of the vagina, which they frequently describe in size as like "an egg," "a lemon," or "an orange." They may also describe pressure or generalized sense of pelvic heaviness. Some may see a bulge when they look at their vulva with a mirror.

Pelvic organ prolapse is not a life-threatening condition, but it may interfere significantly with a woman's quality of life. Mild pelvic organ prolapse may be treated with observation and is checked every year at the annual examination. If the pelvic organ prolapse is bothersome, however, treatment options include a pessary (a silicone disk inserted into the vagina to hold things up, sort of like a diaphragm) or surgery.

99. I am menopausal. Do I still need to see a gynecologist? I have had a hysterectomy. Do I still need a gynecologist?

The health issues that women face beginning at age 50 are different from those they faced when they were younger.

Yes! In the next decade, more women than ever will be 50 years old or older. The health issues that women face beginning at age 50 are different from those they faced when they were younger. Heart disease, osteoporosis, breast cancer, and diabetes occur more often in older women, and some women have higher risks for developing these conditions than others. Furthermore, as your body is going through changes, routine examinations allow you the opportunity to address any questions or concerns you may have. For many women, their gynecologist is their primary care provider.

As women age, screening for health problems becomes increasingly important. Breast cancer is the second most common type (after lung) in women, and colon cancer is third. Gynecologists will perform an annual breast examination on all women. The risk of breast cancer increases with each decade of life, and thus, routine examinations, monthly self-exams, and mammograms are essential. According to the American Cancer Society, women 40 years old or older should have a yearly mammogram.

Depending on your personal history, you may not need a Pap smear every year; instead, you may be able to have one every other or every third year, but this does not mean that you don't need a pelvic examination. Pelvic examinations allow the provider to evaluate internal organs such as the uterus and ovaries for presence or absence of abnormalities. Cancers or premalignant conditions of the vulva or the vagina occur most commonly in postmenopausal women and are readily detected on physical examination. Gynecologists usually perform a rectal examination during the pelvic examination, and many colon cancers are detected in this way. The American Cancer Society recommends a colonoscopy to women who are 50 years and older.

Therefore, an annual pelvic examination gives you and your doctor an opportunity to screen for a variety of diseases, as well as review your overall well-being. For women who have had a hysterectomy (removal of the uterus and cervix), the remaining pelvic tissues, such as the ovaries, if still present, benefit from routine monitoring. Annual pelvic exams can help detect ovarian cancer that may otherwise go undetected; therefore, routine examinations are still beneficial. If no ovaries are present, there is still a small risk of developing a similar condition to ovarian cancer in the tissue that lines all of the pelvic organs, the peritoneum. Thus, you should undoubtedly continue to get examinations.

100. What can I expect in the vulvovaginal region with menopause?

In a premenopausal woman, the vulva and vagina are pink, and the vagina has folds of skin. This is partially due to the effects of estrogen, which helps to ensure a good blood supply to these areas, keeping the tissues healthy and plush. At the time of menopause, when a woman's ovaries stop producing estrogen, a variety of changes may occur, such as irregular vaginal bleeding, cessation of menstruation, hot flashes, and over time vulvovaginal atrophy. Atrophy is the medical term to describe a thinning and weakening of a part of the body. The vagina and vulva which are very sensitive to the effects of estrogen may become atrophic; these areas may become pale or even white, and the walls of the vagina lose their folds of skin and become flat and smooth. Although some women don't notice much of a change, others may experience itching, burning, difficulty lubricating during sexual activity, and pain, especially with intercourse. Also, because the tissues are thinner and not as supple, some women experience more infections, including urinary tract infections. Many women find that even a little bit of estrogen cream alleviates their symptoms. Discuss this with your provider.

Glossary

A

Abscess: A local accumulation of pus that may occur anywhere in the body.

Adenocarcinoma: A malignant tumor of a gland-like structure

Adenosis: The persistence of glands in the vagina that are usually covered over by the vaginal squamous lining in the fetal life.

Aphthae: Another word for a canker sore.

B

Bacteria: A microscopic one-celled organism.

Bacterial vaginosis: Caused by an overgrowth of specific bacteria that normally lives in the vagina. Women frequently describe a "fishy" odor that is particularly strong after intercourse. You cannot get bacterial vaginosis from a toilet seat, bed sheets, or swimming pools.

Bartholin's glands: Paired glands at the 4- and 8-o'clock positions at the vaginal opening. Sometimes they can become infected and form a painful abscess.

Biopsy: A small piece of tissue is removed, usually performed in the office with local anesthesia so that a diagnosis can be made.

C

Candidiasis: Any of a variety of infections caused by fungi of the genus *Candida,* occurring most often in the mouth, respiratory tract, or vagina.

Carcinoma: An invasive malignant tumor derived from epithelial tissue that tends to metastasize to other areas of the body.

Cervix: A part of internal female anatomy that is the lower part of the uterus (womb).

Chancre: The initial lesion of syphilis, commonly a more or less distinct ulcer or sore with distinct edges.

Chancroid: A soft, highly infectious, nonsyphilitic venereal ulcer of the genital region, caused by the bacillus *Hemophilus ducreyi.*

Chemotherapy: The treatment of disease by means of chemicals that have a specific toxic effect or that selectively destroy cancerous tissue.

Chlamydia: A sexually transmitted disease that may be asymptomatic in women or may cause yellow or green vaginal discharge. It is treated with antibiotics. Chlamydia, like gonorrhea, may be associated with pelvic inflammatory disease and infertility.

Clitoral hood: A protective hood of skin that covers the clitoris.

Clitoris: The erectile organ of the female vulva, homologous to the penis of the male.

Colposcope: A magnifying and photographic device used as an aid in the diagnostic examination of the female vulva, vagina, and cervix.

Colposcopy: A procedure where the cervix is visualized with a special microscope called a colposcope. It is a painless outpatient procedure. Sometimes a biopsy is taken at the same time.

Cone biopsy: Refers to a surgical procedure to remove part of the female cervix.

Crohn's disease: A chronic inflammatory disease of the bowel that may cause scarring and thickening of the intestinal walls and frequently leads to obstruction.

Cryotherapy: A method of treating external genital warts by freezing them.

D

Desquamative inflammatory vaginitis: A specific type of vaginitis that is characterized by copious, yellow-green discharge. It is not associated with a specific infecting organism.

Dyspareunia: The medical term for painful sexual intercourse. There are many causes of dyspareunia, and it is a common complaint among women of all ages.

E

Eczema: An inflammatory condition of the skin attended with itching and the exudation of serous matter.

Endometriosis: The presence of endometrial tissue in an incorrect location. In some women, it is associated with pain and infertility. Rarely, it occurs on the vulva.

Episiotomy: Refers to a surgical incision of the perineum to enlarge the vagina and so facilitate delivery during childbirth.

F

Fallopian tubes: A pair of long, slender ducts in the female abdomen that transport ova from the ovary to the uterus and, in fertilization, transport sperm cells from the uterus to the released egg.

Fibroepithelial polyps: Refers to a benign polyp which is a projecting growth from a mucous skin surface.

Folliculitis: Refers to inflammation of hair follicles.

Fomites: Any agent, as clothing or bedding, that is capable of absorbing and transmitting the infecting organism of a disease.

Fordyce spots: Yellow-colored sebaceous glands (skin glands) that are visible through the thin labial skin.

G

Genital herpes: A sexually transmitted disease caused by herpes simplex virus type 1 or 2, characterized primarily by transient blisters on and around the genitals.

Genital warts: A sexually transmitted disease caused by HPV.

Gonorrhea: A sexually transmitted disease which may be asymptomatic in women or may cause yellow or green vaginal discharge. It is treated with antibiotics.

Granuloma fissuratum: Refers to splitting or "fissuring" of the female introitus.

H

Herpes simplex virus: The name of the virus that causes genital herpes.

Hidradenitis suppurativa: An inflammatory condition that affects regions of the body containing sweat glands such as the armpit, under the breasts, in the creases of the thighs, buttocks, and vulva. It is more common in women, particularly those who are obese. Draining pustules, abscesses, blackheads, and swellings ("boils") characterize the condition, which can cause a great deal of distress.

Human papilloma virus: The name of the virus that causes genital warts as well as cervical cancer. There are many different strains of this virus. The strains that cause genital warts are different from the ones that are associated with cancer of the cervix.

Human papilloma virus vaccine: Recently developed to prevent the transmission of certain types of the human papilloma virus, thereby reducing the chances of getting cervical cancer.

Hymen: A fold of mucous membrane partly closing the external orifice of the vagina.

I

Imiquimod: Used to treat external genital and anal warts (***condyloma accuminata***).

Immunosuppression: The inhibition of the normal immune response because of disease, the administration of drugs, or surgery.

Intraepithelial neoplasia: Also known as cervical dysplasia; a potentially premalignant transformation and abnormal growth (dysplasia) of squamous cells on the surface of the cervix.

K

KOH prep: "KOH" is the chemical name for "potassium hydroxide," which is mixed with a small sample of vaginal discharge and examined under a microscope to diagnose a yeast infection.

L

Labia majora (large lips): Two fat pads that are typically covered with pubic hair-bearing skin after puberty. Between the labia majora is the labia minora.

Labia minora (small lips): These are two folds of tissue that meet at the sensitive clitoral hood.

Labioplasty: The name for a medical procedure where the labia minora or majora are made smaller. It is sometimes called a vulvoplasty.

Lactobacilli: A special type of bacteria found normally in the vagina. They maintain a healthy acidic environment in the vagina that inhibits the growth of other "harmful" bacteria and keeps the vagina healthy.

Laryngeal papillomatosis: A condition characterized by multiple squamous cell papillomas of the larynx, seen most commonly in young children, usually due to infection by the human papilloma virus transmitted at birth from the maternal genital warts.

Leiomyoma: Benign tumors of the uterus, also known as "fibroids."

Lichen planus: A rare inflammatory, noninfectious, noncontagious skin disorder that may be found in many areas of the body, including the genitalia and mouth.

Lichen sclerosus: A dermatologic disorder that may affect the vulva. The vulvar skin becomes thin or atrophic, white, and wrinkly, associated with severe itching.

Lichen simplex chronicus: Also called squamous cell hyperplasia; lichen simplex chronicus is a thickening of the vulvar skin that is the result of an uninterrupted cycle of itching and scratching. The more one itches, the more one scratches, which in turn induces more itching.

Local extension: Spread from an organ or tissue to an adjacent one.

Lymphedema: The accumulation of lymph in soft tissue with accompanying swelling, often of the extremities sometimes caused by inflammation, obstruction, or removal of lymph channels.

M

Marsupialization: Refers to the surgical alteration of a cyst by making an incision and suturing the flaps to the adjacent tissue, creating an opening for the cyst to drain.

Melanoma: Any of several types of skin tumors characterized by the malignant growth of melanocytes (pigment forming skin cells).

Menopause: The decrease of estrogen levels in women. A variety of changes may occur including thinning of the vulvar skin. The vulvar skin is sensitive to the effects of estrogen and without it becomes delicate, thin, dry, and sometimes more sensitive.

Metastases: The transference of malignant or cancerous cells to other parts of the body by way of the blood or lymphatic vessels or membranous surfaces.

Micropapillomatosis labialis: Small bumps on the labia minora which are a normal variant and do not represent an infection.

Microtome: An instrument for cutting very thin sections, as of organic tissue, for microscopic examination.

Molluscum contagiosum: A virus disease of the skin marked by round white swellings; transmitted from person to person (most often in children or in adults with impaired immune function).

Mons pubis: A rounded fleshy protuberance situated over the pubic bones that becomes covered with hair during puberty.

N

Neoplasm: A new, often uncontrolled growth of abnormal tissue.

O

Oncologist: A physician who specializes in the treatment of cancer.

Ovarian cysts: Fluid fulled growths in the ovary, which may be related to ovulation, or may reflect a benign or rarely malignant new growth.

Ovaries: The female gonad or reproductive gland, in which the ova and the hormones that regulate female secondary sex characteristics develop.

Oxalate crystal: Oxalate crystals are normal in urine, but in high amounts may contribute to vulvar pain, although this hasn't been established with certainty.

P

Paget's disease: Presents with a very itchy, rashy-looking, red, oozy area on the vulva. It can be thought of as an in-situ cancer, usually, however, it can be associated with adenocarcinomas (cancer of a gland) elsewhere in the body.

Pap smear: Short for "Papanicolaou" test, named after the physician who described taking a sample of cells from a woman's cervix as a way to screen for cervical cancer.

Paraffin block: A wax block. The biopsy is placed in the paraffin block so that thin slices of the biopsy can be made.

Pathologist: A doctor who studies the origin, nature, and course of diseases.

Pelvic inflammatory disease: A term used to describe any infection in the lower female reproductive tract that spreads to the upper female reproductive tract.

Pelvic organ prolapse: Protrusion or descent of any of the female pelvic organs such as the uterus, vagina, bladder, or rectum.

Perineum: The area in front of the anus extending to the fourchette of the vulva in the female.

Pessary: A device worn in the vagina to support a displaced uterus, usually made of silicone or plastic.

Physiologic discharge: Normal vaginal discharge caused by the glands inside the vagina and cervix that make small amounts of fluid that may come out of the vagina. This normal discharge helps to keep the vagina healthy and clean.

Plasma cell vulvitis: Also known as Zoon's vulvitis, this is a rare dermatologic condition that can affect the vulva.

Podofilox: A medication used to treat genital warts.

Podophyllin: A topical medication used to treat external genital warts.

Prophylactic: Preventive or protective.

Psoriasis: A common chronic inflammatory skin disease characterized by scaly patches.

Pubic lice: Small, six-legged parasites that infect the genital hair area and lay eggs.

R

Radiation: The treatment of disease (especially cancer) by exposure to a radioactive substance.

Radical vulvectomy: A surgical procedure performed to treat vulvar cancer. It involves removal of vulvar tissue and is usually combined with resection of the lymph nodes from the groin.

Recombinant: A recombinant vaccine contains a substance that stimulates the immune system without containing viral DNA.

S

Scabies: A contagious skin disease caused by the itch mite, *Sarcoptes scabiei,* which burrows under the skin.

Sentinel lymph nodes: The first lymph nodes a cancer usually spreads to.

Sexually transmitted disease: Also known as "STD" or venereal disease. This term refers to any disease transmitted by sexual contact and is transmitted via semen, vaginal secretions, or blood during intercourse. Sexually transmitted diseases include HIV, chlamydia, genital herpes, genital warts, gonorrhea, syphilis, and some forms of hepatitis.

Squamous cell hyperplasia: An irregular white or gray patch of the skin of the vulva that is slightly raised (thickened).

Staging: A standardized system of determining if a cancer has spread and how advanced a cancer is. It is different for each type of cancer.

Suppression therapy: Therapy to prevent or decrease the number of outbreaks.

Syphilis: A specific sexually transmitted disease which can be associated with a rash in early stages and with neurological impairment in late stages of the disease. In most cases, syphilis can be treated with penicillin.

T

Tinea cruris: A fungal infection of the skin of the groin area, occurring more commonly in warm weather and characterized by red ring-like areas, sometimes with small blisters, and severe itching.

Trichloroacetic acid: Used in a diluted form to treat genital warts.

Trichomonas: A sexually transmitted disease caused by a parasite, *Trichomonas vaginalis*. It often presents with a thin, watery vaginal discharge and itching.

Trichomoniasis: A form of vagintis caused by *Trichomoniasis vaginalis*, it can cause a yellow-green bubble discharge.

U

Urethra: The canal through which urine is discharged from the bladder.

Uterus: The female womb.

V

Vaccine: A substance that stimulates the body's immune response, causing the body to produce disease-preventing or disease-fighting antibodies. The goal of vaccination is to prevent or control an infection. Usually, a specific vaccine is designed to prevent a specific disease.

Vagina: The passage leading from the uterus to the vulva in women.

Vaginitis: Inflammation of the vagina. It may or may not be caused by a sexually transmitted disease.

Verruca vulgaris: The common skin wart.

Vestibular papillomatosis: More prominent thickening and folding of the skin of the labia and can look like bumps. This is due to the increase in hormone levels that occurs during puberty. Vestibular papillomatosis should not be mistaken for human papilloma virus (genital warts); rather, they are a normal finding.

Vestibulodynia: Pain specifically in the vulvar vestibule.

Vulva: A woman's external genitalia. The vulva includes the mons pubis, the clitoris, the inner labia minora (small lips) and labia majora (large lips), and the opening to the vagina (but not the vaginal canal itself), called the vulvar vestibule.

Vulvar cancer: The fourth most common female genital tract cancer and comprises 5% of malignancies of the female genital tract. Squamous cell carcinoma is the most common type of vulvar cancer.

Vulvar intraepithelial neoplasia: A preinvasive carcinoma with no metastatic potential. The incidence of vulvar intraepithelial neoplasia has more than doubled in recent years, particularly in younger women.

Vulvar vestibule: A part of the vulva between the labia minora that the urethral opening and the vaginal opening.

Vulvodynia: Term used for a vulvar pain syndrome, in which the cause is unknown.

Vulvoscopy: A special microscope is used to examine the vulva under high-power visualization. Vulvoscopy is a painless outpatient procedure.

W

Wet mount: Term for a test where a few drops of saline and vaginal discharge are applied to a slide and examined under a microscope.

Y

Yeast infection: Yeast (candida albicans) is a normal inhabitant of the vagina; however, overgrowth of this organism in the vagina may cause vaginal itching and a "cottage cheese"-like discharge. It is not a sexually transmitted disease.

Index

D

E

F

G

H

I

O

P

R

S

T

U

V

W

Y

Z